D0979001

GRAIN OF TRUTH

Also by Stephen Yafa

Cotton: The Biography of a Revolutionary Fiber

GRAIN OF TRUTH

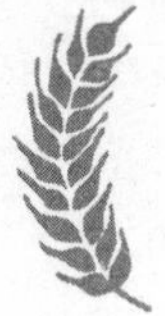

THE REAL CASE FOR AND AGAINST WHEAT AND GLUTEN

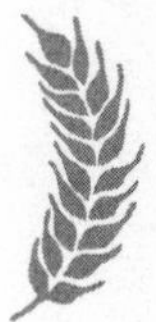

STEPHEN YAFA

AVERY

An imprint of Penguin Random House
375 Hudson Street
New York, New York 10014

Most Avery books are available at special quantity discounts for bulk purchase for sales promotions, premiums, fund-raising, and educational needs. Special books or book excerpts also can be created to fit specific needs. For details, write Special.Markets@penguinrandomhouse.com

LIBRARY OF CONGRESS CATALOGING-IN-PUBLICATION DATA

Yafa, Stephen H., 1941– author.
Grain of truth : the real cause for and against wheat and gluten / Stephen Yafa.
pages cm
Includes bibliographical references and index.
ISBN 978-1-59463-249-5 (hardcover)
1. Gluten-free diet. 2. Wheat-free diet. 3. Wheat. 4. Gluten. I. Title
RM237.86.Y34 2015
633.1'1—dc23 2015005944

Printed in the United States of America
1 3 5 7 9 10 8 6 4 2

Set in New Caledonia
Designed by Eve L. Kirch

To Bonnie, who somehow keeps all our planets from spinning off into space

Contents

GRAIN OF TRUTH

Prologue

One of the many bonds between my wife, Bonnie, and myself has long been the sturdy armor of skepticism we have both erected to protect us from the relentless onslaught of dietary, fashion, lifestyle, and spiritual fads, all directed toward creating a slimmer, bouncier, brighter-eyed, whiter-toothed, higher-functioning you and me—just the sort of evolved being we've both learned to dodge at cocktail parties. Over two decades we'd lived through the Atkins, Pritikin, Scarsdale, South Beach, Blood Type, Beverly Hills, Detox, Israeli Army, Cabbage Soup, and Grapefruit diets and emerged more or less intact. We'd survived break dancing, the Maharishi, Pet Rocks, Rubik's Cubes, Cabbage Patch Dolls, Beanie Babies, ant farms, granny glasses, lava lamps, leisure suits, strobe lights, and Tony Robbins. There have been scars but no damage to major organs including the cerebral cortex—or so I thought.

Then came the Ayurvedic retreat. Bonnie and three female friends disappeared into the hills near Calistoga in Napa County one December morning for a weekend of intense spa treatments. Returning home, my wife made an announcement. "I have a gluten neck," she said. Her first words. I waited for the punch line. None followed. Apparently two male Ayurvedic practitioners, who work on you as a team—I know how this sounds—performed their tandem bodywork on Bonnie. She said she half-expected to be massaged by a guru with a white goatee and a turban. The ancient Indian practice of Ayurvedic medicine, she understood, dates back more than twenty-five hundred years and stresses the balance of three internal *doshas*—water, fire, and air. Beneath the exotic nomenclature is an emphasis on a healthy body-mind connection, a smooth-running metabolism, and an unimpeded digestive system.

"One of the bodyworkers dug his knuckles into the kinks in my neck and shoulders and after a minute he just stopped," Bonnie reported. "He told me, 'There's very little I can do for you until you stop eating gluten. Your upper torso is so inflamed that if you sincerely want to see change, you'll have to take gluten out of your diet.' And I am, starting now." This was not the punch line I expected.

The first items to disappear from our kitchen pantry were pumpernickel, crusty sourdough with its spongy interior, and every other form of wheat-based, chewy, delicious bread and bagel. In their place a whole cast of pretenders moved in like squatters, bearing no resemblance to the authentic original—loaves begging to be called bread yet made from tapioca, rice, sorghum, potato, cornstarch, and flour; crackers and cookies and other assorted dry, brittle wannabe edibles that I snipped off with my front teeth like slivers of seasoned cardboard and attempted to crunch into bite-size units capable of being swallowed. Whether eating non-gluten pizza, pastry, or ersatz pasta, the experience of savoring and chewing anything springy and doughy soon became a nostalgic memory at best, the way that bright sun glows only in dim recollections of characters in bleak postapocalyptic novels. Nothing remained of the heady scent, elasticity, and buoyant texture I associate with leavened wheat. What I'm eating isn't food, I decided: it is punishment for running the occasional red light and sins I've yet to commit.

You may wonder why I didn't stock up on a gluten-rich grain trove of my own in self-defense. Spousal loyalty had something to do with it—Bonnie was committed to her new regimen—but beyond that, I began on my own to investigate the current print, social, and broadcast media assaults on wheat, and they were both voluminous and daunting. Gluten, all agreed, was Satan's spawn. Characterizing wheat as a "healthy whole grain" constitutes "colossally bad advice," Dr. William Davis proclaimed in *Wheat Belly*. It is "among the biggest health blunders ever made in the history of nutritional science." If consuming refined white flour was comparable to smoking unfiltered Camels, he added, eating whole grains was no healthier than inhaling filtered cigarettes.

The basic argument, by now familiar to one and all, goes something like this: gluten, a complex protein found in wheat, rye, and barley, triggers a variety of inflammatory and digestive reactions while the carb content in grain spikes blood glucose and, as a result, promotes insulin resistance, deposits visceral fat, and contributes to obesity, type 2 diabetes, and a host of inflammatory disorders, one of the most severe being celiac disease. That autoimmune reaction in about 1 percent of the population severely damages the small intestine and leaks unwanted bacteria into the blood system. While no cure exists, it can be accurately diagnosed and negative effects can be avoided by refraining from eating wheat, rye, and barley in any form. For the vast majority of us, however, the alleged culprit is non-celiac gluten sensitivity, a more elusive and widespread condition. While it does no damage to our intestinal walls, gluten sensitivity is said to play havoc with our systems in the myriad ways listed above. Hunger cravings, joint pain, and constipation round out gluten's rap sheet.

Closer to home, my wife and dozens of others I talked to, men and women, reported an increase in mental clarity and sustained energy and less bloating as a result of abstaining from wheat. Weight loss figured in, but without the dramatic decreases reported by cardiologist Davis.

While pondering the potential demise of our national grain, planted across fifty million acres of our heartland, I came across a startling statistic. Based on a survey by the marketing research NPD Group, *Time* magazine reported in early 2013 that just under 30 percent of one thousand respondents agreed with the statement: "I'm trying to cut back or avoid gluten in my diet." By extension, that penciled out to about one hundred million Americans who were reducing wheat intake or banishing it from the larder.

What to make of the public's eager willingness to take Davis and company's demonization of the grain as gospel truth? If the non-gluten food phenomenon began as a niche movement a few years earlier, it was now reaching epidemic, critical-mass proportions. To me, wheat had become a grain convicted of bodily harm and sentenced to permanent exile without due process and benefit of counsel. Where exactly was the truth in all this? Who, for instance, was looking at wheat and gluten sensitivity in the larger context of trendy maladies and human nature, not to mention commodity and corporate profits? Having lived through numerous cycles of popular panaceas, I'd come to suspect that you and I are only too ready to take comfort and solace in unearthing a newly discovered source for what ails us, the less likely the better. And what could be less of a potential threat than wheat, the Breakfast of Champions? Who among us would not be thrilled to find relief from the anxiety of not knowing why we feel the way we do, especially if the answer turns out to be as close at hand as a baguette or cereal box? What part, if any, do hard evidence and common sense play in this scenario? My journalistic instincts, I noticed, had after a few weeks become fully engaged. Each new smear provoked an increasing desire on my part to hit the streets, follow leads, and snoop and badger as necessary in order to separate fact from fiction. I wanted to know why an edible as fundamental and ancient as wheat suddenly seemed toxic, and who, if anyone, was standing up for it. That journey took me from a heritage wheat grower in Massachusetts to mass-market wheat fields in Nebraska to a bread lab in Washington State, from a stint as an apprentice baker in Brooklyn to millers in Petaluma to a celiac medical symposium in Chicago to an annual conference for breadheads, and beyond.

Grain of Truth is the result of this effort to explore the true nature of wheat today, absent the hysteria surrounding the grain. Given the unique circumstances of wheat's fall from grace as a wholesome, healthful food product, this book also looks at how that reversal of fortune is playing out among the country's largest wheat-based industries. At no time in our history has a major food staple endured such widespread public distrust. Wheat has become *granum non grata* from Whole Foods in Beverly Hills to mom-and-pop grocery shops in the blue-collar neighborhoods of Staten Island, where I've come upon tattered awnings prominently advertising the non-gluten, wheat-free selections within. If you're the wheat industry, I wondered, what do you do? Do you simply hunker down and wait for a backlash against the gluten backlash, or do you mount an aggressive public relations campaign to counter the avalanche of bad publicity?

Companies like Post Foods and Pepperidge Farm seemed at first glance to be operating in an alternate universe. Entering "gluten" into the search field on their websites produced a one-line response: "Sorry, there are no results that match what you searched for." Others, like General Mills and Kellogg's, produced such offerings as "Chex-gluten-free" or "New Gluten-Free Rice Krispies," a staggering three hundred–plus non-gluten products from GM alone. Does that qualify as a capitulation to current opinion without a peep of protest? None seemed willing to defend wheat, bravely and boldly or even meekly, although traditionally it has comprised a significant share of their business. I sensed that somewhere cereal scientists were delving into the composition of gluten's amino-acid mysteries looking for ways to neutralize the molecule's most problematic properties. Little did I know I would indeed discover that research—in Italy.

I saw my investigative charge quite simply as probing where necessary and seeking out experts—wheat growers, millers, bakers, bioscientists, nutritionists, and physicians—with credentials and insights that could be trusted to add perspective and help ferret out telling details that Davis and others possibly overlooked or chose to ignore. I quickly realized that there was much more to the story that remained yet untold. As one example, that long fermentation—the action of yeast and lactobacilli on flour that produces leavened sourdough—can play a crucial role in breaking down gluten proteins to make them more easily digestible and less disruptive. I also learned, much to my delight, that by focusing on white flour derived from nitrogen-boosted commodity grain, wheat's detractors skipped over the best part of the story, the remarkable array of flavors and tastes—as well as nutritional benefits—that wheat delivers when bred, farmed, and processed by local artisans to accentuate its strengths. An entire library of heritage wheats goes unexplored by the mainstream industry. And I trusted myself to tell the tale of wheat as an American icon. For all but the past few years this grain has been on a mythological hero's journey. It has fueled Olympic gold medalists and All-Stars who did exactly what their mothers told them to do: Eat your Wheaties! Amber waves of grain figure into the country's saga as indelibly as the soaring bald eagle, the Alamo, or Betsy Ross's stars and stripes. Nothing is as American as apple pie, and apple pie itself is nothing without the flaky wheat crust that caresses the warm, cinnamon-scented fruit filling from below and spans it from above in a latticework of diamond-shaped bands of golden baked wheat dough.

Every copper penny through 1958 displayed a profile of Lincoln on its front and two wheat stalks on its reverse side. While both the president and the grain were instrumental in shaping the destiny of our country, those shafts alone symbolized prosperity, robust health, and thrift all at once—fundamental American goals and accepted virtues. It seemed only fitting that I keep a Lincoln penny in my pocket as I set out to explore wheat's economic and cultural heritage and its future prospects in turbulent times. These days a penny can't buy much, but this one inspired the kind of passionate curiosity that to me ranks as a currency beyond measure.

What's Up with Wheat?

History celebrates the battlefield whereon we meet our death, but scorns to speak of the plowed fields whereby we thrive; it knows the names of kings' bastards but cannot tell us the origin of wheat. That is the way of human folly.

—Jean-Henri Fabre
French Entomologist

I'm still eating my Wheaties. That may single me out as the last man standing in America who isn't smart enough to avoid belly fat, premature dementia, skin rashes, stiff joints, insulin resistance, and a leaky gut by not giving up wheat. Eating that All-American cereal grain once marked me as a health-conscious guy intent on toning his muscles, slimming down, and adding the fiber that we all need to benefit digestion and elimination. Today it defines me as clueless and out of touch with some current medical and nutritionist thinking about the perils of ingesting what has come to be seen as a dangerous grain. Either I'm someone who chooses to ignore wheat's allegedly hazardous starch and gluten content, or I'm just a lunkhead who keeps up with the latest health guidance bulletins only to reject their advice.

I see it a little differently. In fact, I'm puzzled that something as fundamental as wheat, a food source we've consumed for at least ten thousand years, suddenly seems toxic. It provides about 20 percent of the world's calories, as much as 45 percent of daily protein in many developing countries, and nourishes more people on earth than any other food. For better than a year I explored the world of American wheat and came away convinced that it isn't the grain, it's the way we grow and process it from seed to shelf that determines whether wheat supports or jeopardizes our basic health needs. That includes the methods used by farmers to fertilize and protect their plants from pests and weeds in the field and by our nation's large wheat-product manufacturers to transform the dried seeds into flour and then dough before baking. Nobody wants to hear that human intervention more than any other factor might be the source of the problem, if indeed there is one, with wheat, not when gluten-free products are predicted to rack up more than $15 billion in sales by 2016. But that's exactly the case. We've done a masterful job of designing machinery that feeds us the worst of wheat while stripping off the best of it, the plant's nutritious components, for animal feed.

Scared Witless

More on that to come, but first, a closer look at the bad rap on wheat. It's understandable that anyone browsing the Internet, picking up a magazine, roaming a bookstore, chatting with neighbors or friends over a latte, or tweeting online would come away with severe cereal paranoia. The assault has been relentless and, while various grains are culprits, wheat has been targeted because its seeds, or kernels, contain much more gluten than rye or barley, the two other grains with the same protein. Gluten, which provides food storage for the germinating seed, is actually a complex comprised of two amino-acid proteins, gliadin and glutenin, that bond to form long, tangled molecules. Its stickiness—*gluten* comes from the Latin word for "glue"—adds elasticity and extensibility to wheat flour when mixed with water. The cohesion enables kneaded dough to stretch and hold its shape, a delicate compromise between strength and flexibility that gluten alone provides.

Bakers, for that reason, depend on gluten to create structure and resilience in their bread doughs. With the addition of water, this amino-acid bead string produces a web matrix of dough, the crumb. Carbon dioxide, the escaping gas released as a yeast by-product, fills the air pockets—named alveoli, like the lung's balloon-like structures. That causes the crumb to swell inside the rising crust as it bakes. "Gluten," Michael Pollan has observed, "is the reason that wheat was able to conquer the planet." But we're not bakers, most of us, we're baked goods consumers, scared witless by the barrage of bad press surrounding these gluey molecules and the glucose-laden carbohydrate starch surrounding them.

As might be predicted, many of the country's most famous and lauded chefs, including Mario Batali and the Michelin multi-starred super chef Thomas Keller, whose gastronomical empire ranges from The French Laundry in Napa to Per Se in New York to Bouchon at the Venetian in Las Vegas, have eagerly embraced the movement. Keller and one of his prizewinning pastry chefs created Cup4Cup, a gluten-free tapioca, brown rice, and potato flour blend sold at Williams-Sonoma at $20 for three pounds, a king's ransom.

According to a restaurant survey quoted in a *New Yorker* article, in 2013 we ordered more than two hundred million gluten-free or wheat-free dishes. We didn't do that to enhance our enjoyment of flavor and texture. We did it more or less for the same reason that gluten-free dog biscuits—"keep veggie-loving pup tails waggin'"—now call up over two million search results on Google, that gluten-wary couples now use separate toaster and butter knives, and that gluten-free ocean cruises have gained a loyal following.

We've been poleaxed by doomsday messages that warn us away from all things glutenized, not subtly or with qualifications. William Davis in *Wheat Belly* asserts that wheat has been "destroying more brains in this country than all the strokes, car accidents and head trauma combined." "The perfect poison," he calls it. "Eating wheat, like ice climbing, mountain boarding, and bungee jumping, is an extreme sport. It is the only common food that carries its own long-term mortality rate." In his best seller, *Grain Brain*, Dr. David Perlmutter claims that 40 percent of us cannot properly process gluten, and the remaining 60 percent may be in harm's way.

But fear alone does not persuade so effectively without a reward for compliance, and in this instance it's the promise of weight loss. Lose the wheat, lose the weight. Books and blogs are crammed with testimonials, as in this excerpt that Dorothy, eighteen pounds lighter, posted on *The Daily Dietribe*: "OMG, I really can't believe it. I understood immediately, this Gluten Free Challenge is going to save my life. It's going to take me from 'surviving life' to living life again. It may even change my career path." As might be expected, the non-gluten expo and festival business is booming across the country. Wherever you live there is likely to be an event within a few weeks and a day's jaunt from your home, whether in West Palm Beach or Dallas, Ottawa or Calgary, Atlanta or Indianapolis, as well as scores of cities in between at all times of the year. Major markets are not the only venues. More than six thousand folks showed up at a one-day expo in Sandy, Utah, funded by General Mills, to chow down an enormous gluten-free pancake breakfast. Just about every food chain and food-and-entertainment enterprise in America today creates a special menu that caters to the wheatless. Disney's Liberty Tree Tavern at Magic Kingdom features a gluten-free version of the Pilgrim's Feast for Thanksgiving served in its Betsy Ross room. At last count there were close to a thousand gluten-free cookbooks listed on Amazon.

Probable Cause

Until a decade ago, hardly anyone outside the medical community knew anything about gluten intolerance and celiac disease, the severe autoimmune reaction to gluten that damages the intestinal lining; within that community the condition also remained largely unknown, even among many gastroenterologists. Today, when gluten intolerance has become a common talk-show topic, celebrities line up on both sides and launch verbal grenades at one another. The maxim that you are what you eat has been replaced by a gluten-free postscript. You are what you *don't* eat.

While total intolerance to gluten has been on the rise for past fifty years, celiac disease is still too rare, affecting 1 in 133 or less than 1 percent of the general population, to ignite this phenomenon on its own. People who count themselves as victims of gluten may experience abdominal and joint pain, fatigue, fogginess, bloating, diarrhea, and headaches—symptoms of celiac disease but absent the intestinal lining damage that leads to life-threatening malnutrition.

Those much more common complaints have been linked to non-celiac gluten sensitivity, NCGS.

Unlike celiac disease, for which there are biomarkers, or reliable indicators, gluten sensitivity has yet to show up in any surefire diagnosable form in medical tests. For the time being that leaves self-diagnosis as the only other option. While experts do not discount the connection between probable cause and effect, there is still no firm data. A comprehensive clinical study at the University of Maryland found that 6 percent of patients—347 of 5,896—waiting to be seen at the university hospital self-reported gluten-sensitivity symptoms. Through 2014, this was the most reliable information on its frequency.

Guesswork still trumps blood work. Given all the media and popular attention, I was surprised to discover the science on sensitivity to be more confusing than enlightening. To complicate matters, a year or so ago another country was heard from, as my grandfather might have remarked. Its official name is FODMAPS, which I choose to call Fodmaps because, well, talking or writing in ALL CAPS seems rude. I'll spare you any long-winded explanation for the moment and pick up the subject again after a closer look at gluten intolerance—celiac disease—and gluten sensitivity, but it's worth pointing out that a growing number of medical researchers now believe some symptoms associated with sensitivity may in fact emanate from the carbohydrates found in dozens of fruits and vegetables as well as wheat and other grains. Those sugars, or Fodmaps, an acronym for fermentable oligosaccharides, disaccharides, monosaccharides, and polyols, are poorly digested and may cause many if not all of the intestinal problems ascribed to gluten sensitivity.

I see your eyes glazing over, so enough at present. Who needs a long cheat sheet? We're Americans. We want a quick-fix, one-stop, silver-bullet diet. If it involves a dollop of self-sacrifice, so be it, as long as it leaves the steak on the plate and doesn't require memorizing a dictionary-length list of verboten foods.

That's gluten. One word, three grains, no homework. We can do that. And indeed we do: about one in three of us buys into the idea that a life without wheat in it is a life worth living, especially when we can drop pounds and count celebs like Russell Crowe, Oprah, Lady Gaga, Gwyneth Paltrow, Miley Cyrus, and Novak Djokovic on our side.

But don't show up with a platter of gluten-free brownies at the homes of two leading actresses, Jennifer Lawrence and Charlize Theron, both ardent campaigners for real food, carbs, and gluten included. Theron told talk-show host Chelsea Handler, "I just think that if you are gonna send a gift, let it be enjoyable. Why send me a fucking cupcake with no sugar in it? What's the use? There's no use. It tastes like cardboard!" And Lawrence raised more than a few hackles when she weighed in during a *Vanity Fair* interview on the gluten-free epidemic. She called it "the new, cool eating disorder."

Eating a daily regimen of my own gluten-rich sourdough bread resulted in perfect health, dropped weight, high sustained energy, and a feeling of satiation without bloating. My personal takeaway—and eventually my wife's as well—is that I more or less blundered into a life-changing writing project. It propelled me to investigate and befriend a food source that nourishes, slims, energizes, and tastes great: sourdough breads. I'm getting ahead of myself slightly, I know, but just enough to let you know there is indeed a silver lining in the Jennifer Lawrence pro-gluten playbook, and its name is long-fermented dough.

The Human Factor

At a slightly higher level of discourse, or not, the anti-gluten medical contingent continues to wade in. All lines between professional probity and media hucksterism have long been erased. William Davis regularly shows up as a cruise ship headliner and in Dr. Oz's Kitchen. Neurologist David Perlmutter takes over a ninety-minute PBS special, *Brainchange*, which "blows the lid off a topic that's been buried in medical literature for far too long: carbs are destroying your brain." Wheat, he argues, stimulates the formation of inflammatory cytokines—molecular message proteins that block production of critical neurotransmitters like serotonin. We're lucky if we can still put sentences together.

A regular columnist at the *Huffington Post*, Mark Hyman, MD, claims that wheat contains a "super drug, super gluten and super starch" that drive "obesity, diabetes, heart disease, cancer, dementia and more." He promotes corrective shakes and snacks and detox diets that, no coincidence, he sells at his Healthy Living Store on the Internet. Hyman caught the public's attention when he labeled anything with wheat in it—about one third of all the products in a supermarket—"Frankenfoods."

Is it possible that so many experts, supported by abundant scientific references in their books and speaking with such conviction and certainty, can be wrong?

Absolutely. For the first few months of my research I bought into their full-throttle assaults, then slowly but surely I became aware that they weren't telling me the whole truth. The critical flaw, I learned, is not so much what these medical and other authorities have to say but what they leave out of their arguments.

Us. Our involvement. In whole form, a wheat kernel is no health menace except to celiacs. We've created a huge milling and baking industry that produces refined flour with so little nutritional value that vitamins and minerals have to be injected back into it, yet industrial milling gets no mention in the index of *Wheat Belly* and other broadsides. While wheat was first domesticated from wild grass in an area that extends from Syria to Turkey, the Fertile Crescent, at least ten thousand years ago and probably long before that, not until the last quarter of the nineteenth century did technology become available to quickly and efficiently strip off the outer coat of the seed, the fibrous bran, and the seed's embryo, its germ, in order to mill white flour in massive quantities from its starchy center, or endosperm. Throughout history white endosperm flour has always been favored for its powdery texture, versatility, and easy digestion. Since the absence of lipids, or fats, greatly prolongs its shelf life, white flour—unlike whole-grain—has been equally valued for its durability. For that reason in the days before refrigeration it became a vital food source on wagon trains and long ocean voyages. That engineering breakthrough led to the production of commercial white bread at low cost, available to one and all and until then an unaffordable luxury; food manufacturers sold it with little or no awareness of the grave health consequences it presented to consumers.

Not until World War II, sixty years later, were measures taken to address the vitamin and mineral deficiencies caused by these grain-milling methods. They caught the government's attention only when 40 percent of the raw recruits drafted by our military proved to be so malnourished that they could not pass a physical and were declared unfit for duty. Nutritionists pointed to empty-calorie white bread as a primary cause as they had for decades, without making inroads. Before long, an enrichment protocol was put into practice.

Commercial dough today is routinely loaded with conditioners and additives designed to shortcut natural processes and to function effortlessly with the machines that produce it. In the blink of an eye, fast fermentation transforms flour into packaged loaves and rolls. Industrial bakers now add a potent form of gluten—the powdered concentrate called vital gluten—to thousands of foods from cookies to cakes to lunch snacks and cosmetic products as a binder and thickener. It strengthens dough and helps to precipitate a quick rise of bread as it ferments, which accounts for its wide usage. If we're eating more gluten than ever, as we are, it is because manufacturers have upped the dosage. Breeding experts I talked to report that despite claims to the contrary, modern wheat does not contain an increased percentage of gluten in its endosperm.

Wheat's most vocal adversaries argue that it does and that the gluten proteins have mutated over the last sixty years—frightening assertions, to be sure. On closer inspection, I found these assertions to be based on sketchy evidence that respected scientists in the field dismiss. Wheat's enemies also ignore an approach to growing, processing, and baking that improves its appeal and its health benefits. They do not take into account fresh whole-grain alternatives available in specialty chains like Whole Foods. Those sourdough and other baked goods, created by a burgeoning local artisan community around the country, contain a full complement of nutritive components and fiber. Many consumers with gluten sensitivity complaints report that they eat these products and experience no negative reaction, not a surprise since scientific studies show that microbes produced by long sourdough fermentation, the artisan approach, prove effective in breaking down and neutralizing gluten molecules.

These breads and pastries also belie the notion that 100 percent whole wheat is too dense and bitter to be palatable.

In later chapters I'll circle back to the artisan movement from field to store shelf. For now, the simple point to be made is that the subject is glossed over by the death-to-gluten hit squads. I learned again and again during my research that the way our bodies respond to wheat has everything to do with how we cultivate and process it, for better or worse.

Soldiers of Science

Whether or not justified, wheat bashing has become a national sport. You have to shout above the roar of the crowd in these cacophonous times to be heard, which pretty much rules out wheat's defenders. They tend to go about their business quietly as medical professionals, researchers, and academics offering thoughtful analysis in technical, often turgid papers, away from the spotlight. Unlike Davis, they don't generally pepper their oratory with memorably vivid figures of speech, as in equating wheat eating to bungee jumping or cigarette smoking. It's Fox News versus PBS, and we all know who gets the higher ratings. But these are the soldiers of science who do the unglamorous work of probing into our microbial universe to explore connections and determine verifiable cause-and-effect relationships. One in particular, Julie Miller Jones, professor emerita of food and nutrition at St. Catherine University in Minneapolis–St. Paul, looked over the brief against wheat as presented in the popular press and came away so dismayed by misstatements in *Wheat Belly* that she put together a twenty-two-page, point-by-point refutation of the book's central arguments. She supported her analysis with 116 references.

Unless you subscribe to *Cereal Foods World*, you are unlikely to have come upon it. These journals, with limited circulation, rarely get noticed outside a small community of fellow health professionals. Jones, an LN (licensed nutritionist) who specializes in cereal grains and advises the US Department of Agriculture (USDA), surgically dissected *Wheat Belly*'s core arguments. "The facts Davis presents about central obesity are true and warrant concern," she wrote. "What is not true is that wheat causes this condition and the elimination of wheat will cure this condition."

As one among many examples, she lays waste to Davis's assertion that wheat is "the world's most destructive dietary ingredient" because during digestion it breaks down into peptides, short chains of amino-acid proteins, that "bind to the brain's morphine receptor, the very same receptor to which opiate drugs bind." He calls them exorphins, as in external endorphins. As such, he claims, they cause compulsive hunger urges—an uncontrollable appetite for more of the same carbs that are sending us to an early grave—and they trigger withdrawal symptoms when withheld. Wheat, he adds, is unique among foods in creating that addiction.

Not so, says Jones, among many others. Davis is citing thirty-five-year-old research performed on cell tissue cultures that ascribed exactly the same opium-like effects to milk, soy, spinach, and rice. The researchers treated mouse organs directly with purified opiods, a process not related to consuming and digesting food. No human subjects were involved. Further gut-brain feedback studies, not mentioned by Davis, came to exactly the opposite conclusion, that these foods produce a sensation of fullness, not hunger. A research group at Maastricht University in the Netherlands, publishing in the *Journal of Cereal Science*, jumped all over Davis's contention that your wheat-addicted brain programs you to eat 400 more calories over two meals in order to restimulate those feelings of euphoria.

Said the Dutch scientists: "There is no data available to substantiate this suggestion." They titled their exhaustive overview, "Does Wheat Make Us Fat or Sick?" Their resounding answer: no and no.

Appearing on *CBS This Morning* to make his opium-like-addiction case to Charlie Rose, Davis incited the wrath of Dr. Stefano Guandalini, founder and medical director of the Celiac Disease Center at the University of Chicago and one of the country's leading experts in the field. Guandalini took to Facebook to denounce Davis for basing his evidence on unreliable, dated experiments conducted only on rodents. He criticized CBS for not allowing a qualified expert—like, well, Guandalini himself—to debate the cardiologist on camera, for which he got blasted at once on the Wheat Belly blog. "Among the most ignorant about wheat? Celiac experts!" Davis headlined his blistering counterattack.

But just when it seemed that these two were about to square off on a special doc-versus-doc edition of *WWE Friday Night SmackDown*, Guandalini bowed out. A few months later in conversation at the International Celiac Disease Symposium he hosted in Chicago, he told me that he made that decision because he couldn't afford the time; he had more important things to do. Davis, by contrast, was pumped for a public brawl.

Your Brain on Gluten?

One of the first things I wanted to clear up with Jones when we spoke was any potential conflict of interest. I noted that she is also listed as a scientific adviser to the Grain Foods Foundation, funded by the American baking industry. Was she being paid to take on Davis?

"No. I tell [the foundation] when data says there is a problem that they need to be concerned about," she responded. "I am there to give good nutritional advice. Throughout my career I have tried to bust nutrition myths and fads and promote general good diets. For *Wheat Belly*, I tried to be as dispassionate as possible."

In her paper she points out that Davis makes some right calls. Wheat, as he says, is an allergen. Baker's asthma—caused by the constant presence of flour particles in the air—has been known since Roman times. Allergies are frequently related to the seed storage proteins in gluten. Carbohydrates do indeed increase small, dense LDL (low-density-lipoprotein) cholesterol particles, a potential cardiovascular disease risk, and removal of gluten may reduce the rate of type 1 diabetes.

But, she said, "what really *kills* me with this diet is that it asks people to give up an important source of fiber in wheat bran. As it is, only 4 percent of Americans meet the recommended daily requirement for dietary fiber, and if you're a male between fourteen to fifty, not even 1 percent. I can take any chronic disease endpoint that plagues us—coronary disease, type 2 diabetes, metabolic syndrome, hypertension—and if I compare those people with high fiber intake with those who are at the average of less than half an ounce, your risk of all those diseases and total mortality is reduced by at *least* 20 percent. The data are overwhelming. One of the things fiber does is control the release of glucose into the bloodstream so you don't see those spikes in blood sugar."

Miller's point is taken up in another context by pediatrician and medical geneticist Ayala Laufer-Cahana. "What Davis left out," she says, "is that glycemic load matters much more than any glycemic index number—that is, how much of the food you're eating, and if you're eating it by itself. You're more likely to consume bread as part of a larger meal, with numerous other servings of food, so you're substantially lowering its glycemic load, and slowing the rate of absorption into your bloodstream. On the other hand, if you're drinking a soda you're drinking pretty much pure sugar; 80-plus percent of it is glucose. There's a significant difference." Dr. Ayala, as she's known to her *Huffington Post* readers, reserves most of her anger for Davis's "sweeping polemic against something so central as bread to our culture" without any real proof. His book, she says, is "baseless."

"Cultivating edible grain like wheat is probably one of the most important things in the development of the modern human. If not for that we'd still be hunting and gathering. In many ways it's one of the most miraculous things that people ever invented."

It's a reasonable guess that Jones, an animated, down-to-earth woman with an engaging laugh, would agree. The scientific details of her rebuttal I'll spare you. Her strongest argument is that Davis, not the first scientist to play loose with facts, cherry-picks and distorts research papers to build his case. She leans on her years spent working with obese patients to make a convincing argument that calorie reduction in general, not the removal of wheat or any other single ingredient from a diet, helps cure many of the conditions from rashes to diabetes that medical authors link solely to gluten.

David Perlmutter in *Grain Brain*, meanwhile, takes a position even more extreme than Davis. He likens eating gluten to drinking gasoline and charges wheat with escalating a host of medical problems. He cites a *New England Journal of Medicine* article in which a researcher concludes, "Higher glucose levels may be a risk factor in dementia" and transforms that instantly into "Brain dysfunction starts in your daily bread, and I'm going to prove it. I'll state it again because I know it sounds absurd: Modern grains are silently destroying your brain." He indicts all grains—whole, multigrain, stone-ground, sprouted.

What Davis and Perlmutter share, aside from a large readership, is an aversion to 15-mile-an-hour reduced speed zones when they're thundering down the Diatribe Autobahn at 140 mph to drive home their points. They don't slow for debatable evidence or brake for inconvenient truths. This petal-to-the-metal approach ticks off scores of health professionals who spend much of their time and talent creeping inch by inch through complex, often inconclusive data to search out science that can stand up to close scrutiny, all in an effort to help their patients.

Straddling media and medicine with agility is Dr. David Katz, a leading integrative medical practitioner and founding director of the Yale University Prevention Research Center. In an article in *The Atlantic* by Dr. James Hamblin, "This Is Your Brain on Gluten," Katz lays into Perlmutter: "I also find it sad that because his book is filled with a whole bunch of nonsense, that's why it's a bestseller; that's why we're talking. Because that's how you get on the bestseller list. You promise the moon and stars, you say everything you heard before was wrong, and you blame everything on one thing. You get a scapegoat; it's classic." Katz told me after the article was published that he's worked with Perlmutter and respects him as a physician, but that there is no substance to his arguments.

Foggy-Brained Glutenites

The GF (gluten-free) insignia itself has leapt over semantic boundaries by now to become code language for the trim-at-heart. In a

New Yorker cartoon a woman tells her friend over lunch, "I've only been gluten-free for a week but I'm already annoying."

When people announce minutes after we've been introduced at a dinner party that they're gluten-free, I get the feeling they expect me to applaud and congratulate them for being sleek specimens willing to forgo every pleasure from Cronuts, that mash-up of croissant and doughnut, to linguine vongole in pursuit of a healthier, thinner, laser-brained persona. But they've picked the wrong guy. It's against my nature as a die-hard Triscuit junkie to trash wheat and praise virtuous behavior like excessive self-discipline. Instead I'm more apt to goad them.

"What exactly *is* gluten?" I ask.

"Oh, you know, it's the thing in wheat that makes you fat," I'm most likely to get back as a response.

"But isn't that the carb content? Gluten isn't a carb, it's a protein."

"Oh, well, then it's . . . believe me, I'm never going anywhere near it again, ever, and so shouldn't you."

Most of the time I back off, but every so often, and more often more recently, I run into someone so smug and clueless that I pull out my iPhone and play a now-classic Jimmy Kimmel clip. "A lot of people don't eat gluten because someone in their yoga class told them not to," Kimmel tells his late-night audience by way of introducing the "Pedestrian Question" segment. "I keep wondering, how many of these people even know what gluten is?" To find out, his woman on the street interviews young males and females at a nearby gym who all maintain a gluten-free diet.

"What is gluten?" she asks.

"This is sad," responds the first young guy, bare-chested under a Kansas City baseball cap, "but I really don't know." The next bare-chested guy tells her, "It's a flour derivative, yeah, like bread, like pastries." Pressed for a specific answer, he adds, "It's a grain, right?" And so it goes. The last guy tells her, "It is a part of the wheat, that . . ."—he shakes his head—"Dunno."

My takeaway is that the non-gluten lifestyle has become such a cool, hip statement so divorced from its granular origins that wheat left the building long ago and nobody noticed.

In case you're approached, gluten is the elastic protein package in wheat, rye, and barley that enables bread to swell and hold its domed shape without collapsing. The bead-like gliadin molecules and rope-like glutenins form a network within the dough that traps and holds gas, and allows bread to maintain its shape after it rises. In the plant, as mentioned, gluten provides nourishment as the seed develops a root system and later grows into a seedling. There is no doubt that some of us non-celiacs who are otherwise healthy cannot comfortably digest gluten, but that number—between 1 and 6 percent—bears little relation to the one hundred million of us who think we're better off eliminating or reducing wheat from our diet. The hard evidence suggests that wheat's foes have oversimplified health issues and unnerved a jittery, overwrought public.

For a point of comparison I wanted to learn more about the symptoms people experience when they're not in that self-reported gluten-intolerant zone, but certifiably gluten-intolerant—when any amount of gluten above 20 parts per million is likely to set off a debilitating series of autoimmune reactions. I'd read about the devastation it causes but I'd met no one whom I knew to be victimized by celiac disease, and so I took myself to the annual International Celiac Disease Symposium in Chicago.

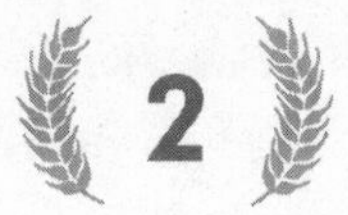

Gut Issues

From the gut comes the strut . . .

—François Rabelais

I knew that many of America's leading medical experts would be at the gathering, as well as many in the audience eager to hear the latest research on their celiac condition. I first tracked down Dr. Alessio Fasano, former director of the University of Maryland Center for Celiac Research; Fasano headed up the original study that put the gluten-sensitivity figure at 6 percent of the general population and is widely considered to be one of the prominent physicians in the field. He'd previously spoken to me from his office in Mass-General Hospital in Boston, where he now works. When we finally met up between conference sessions I asked why, in the span of a few months from our first conversation, the gluten-free movement seemed to be exploding.

He practically snorted in response. "I can give you twenty-five thousand reasons why people more and more hear if they just stop eating wheat they'll suddenly get healthy. The placebo effect, of course. But more important, if you eliminate gluten from your diet, your lifestyle will change dramatically. You'll get much closer to the eating habits of our grandparents. To do it right, you can't eat processed food anymore. Your pain and bloat problems might not even be from gluten but from the fat and simple sugars in our Western diet. You can't shove something frozen in the microwave and call that cooking. Once you begin to eat and cook fresh foods—meat, fish, vegetables, and so on—are you going to feel better? What do you think? Of course. To say that gluten is the enemy of mankind, it's ridiculous!"

All this delivered in a melodic Italian accent, so quickly the words gush like white-water rapids down a narrow shoot. I could see why Fasano has become a go-to media resource. He's peppery, good-looking, effusive, and he knows his stuff. His team in fact first identified non-celiac gluten sensitivity and named it. He is convinced it exists and that in time blood tests—including checking for the presence of positive IgG antigliadin antibodies—will diagnose it as reliably as cholesterol levels. But Fasano is a realist, not an alarmist.

"At the moment there is no certainty in the test results we get. Of course there's such a thing as a non-celiac reaction," he tells me, "and gluten is definitely a tricky molecule that's hard for some to digest, but only for a handful. It came along late in our evolution, ten thousand years ago, and we don't all adapt the same. For some of us it's bound to be problematic. We're still exploring what we don't know, which remains more than what we do. But we'll get there."

Celiac specialist Dr. Stefano Guandalini, who was hosting the downtown Sheraton Towers conference (with thousands from around the globe in attendance), later offered me his own perspective: "I compared the consumption of wheat in Italy with the United States. Italians eat more than twice as much wheat per capita, mostly as pasta. But while we have a 36 percent obesity rate, there is only an 8.3 percent rate in Italy. If gluten is responsible for our obesity epidemic, as Davis in *Wheat Belly* claims, how is it that we have more than four times as many obese people? That's not his hypothesis or mine, but a fact."

Up Close and Personal

Bombarded daily with gluten-related questions, Fasano and Guandalini keep their main focus on treating patients with the much more extreme, definable, and debilitating celiac condition. By contrast to gluten sensitivity, specific genetic biomarkers confirm the presence of celiac disease, first named (*koilliaskos*, or "abdomen") by the Greek physician Aretaeus of Cappadocia in the second century CE. A genetic autoimmune reaction to gluten that, as mentioned, affects 1 in 133, or about 1.8 million Americans (the same 0.9 percentage holds true for populations around the world), celiac disease results from the immune system's misguided attempt to fight off a phantom foreign invader. Like an infantry squadron following the orders of a deranged commanding officer, antibodies attack and destroy the small intestine's fingerlike villi that line the gut wall. If fully functional, they absorb nutrients and pass them into the bloodstream, but in celiacs, when even the smallest amounts of gluten cause the villi to collapse, severe malnutrition and energy loss result, along with a host of related afflictions. Under a microscope the flattened villi resemble grass sprouts leveled by Roundup.

For me, that autoimmune reaction remained an abstract concept until I met up with several former celiac sufferers at the Chicago symposium. One man I talked to, Ethan, now in his late forties, was so fatigued for years that he couldn't work for more than a couple of hours at a time without lying down. Finally—after a decade of incorrect diagnoses, he tested positive for the telltale celiac HLA antigen, completely eliminated gluten from his diet, and gained back all the weight, energy, and strength he'd lost over two decades. "You have no idea what it's like to have to wonder if you can climb five stairs," he told me, "or to have to sit on the top step to catch your breath." He showed me an earlier image of himself as a celiac sufferer that he'd carried around on his iPhone. The man who stared back at the lens was so emaciated, I would never have recognized him as the man across from me.

Ethan's reply surprised me when I asked him what he did for a living. He told me he was a practicing pathologist. "As a physician studying diseases, how come it took so long to make the discovery about yourself?" I wondered.

"I listened to my gastroenterologist," he said. "He tested for everything else, all negative, until celiac started to make itself known in the medical community a few years back and we ordered up blood work. There it was, the biomarker! My future changed almost overnight."

The wife of another physician from North Carolina, Fiona, told me that her daughter, Chloe, fell into such a deep depression as a teenager that she was on suicide watch, that no antidepressants helped, that at her darkest moments she could barely get out of bed. By chance, Fiona heard two women discussing gluten intolerance over coffee at Starbucks. She had Chloe tested for the genetic markers, and once gluten was removed from Chloe's diet, she improved so rapidly that she was able to go off to college on her own two months later.

Numerous other encounters with celiacs or family members over the two days of the conference generated much of the same and led me to a simple conclusion: this disease is the worst kind of monster; if undiagnosed it hides in plain sight and slowly, corrosively, and relentlessly saps out all vitality, leaving you a shell of your former self.

Puzzling Increase

As with many other genetic conditions, I learned at the symposium, celiac disease follows no predictable script. Roughly 30 percent of people with European ancestry carry predisposing genes, for example. Yet more than 95 percent of the carriers tolerate gluten just fine. For some it remains dormant until a grilled cheese sandwich or slice of toast suddenly—and mysteriously—activates the inflammatory autoimmune response, from which point on the individual cannot tolerate gluten.

Joseph A. Murray, an acclaimed expert on celiac disease and a medical professor at the Mayo Clinic, discovered that blood samples had been saved from nine thousand US Air Force recruits in the year immediately following World War II. He assumed that close to 1 percent—as at present—would carry antibodies to a specific body-repairing enzyme, which is a biomarker for celiac disease. (The most common test looks for elevated levels of a telltale antibody, IgA, which frequently attacks that enzyme, tTG, in celiac sufferers.)

Instead his team found the antibody originally in only two tenths of 1 percent of those recruits, leading Murray to conclude that celiac disease has doubled every fifteen years in the past half century and is now four times more prevalent for reasons that no one has been able to determine with any certainty. Because the increase affects young and old alike, he and others suspect that the cause may be environmental.

Research scientist Stephanie Seneff, at MIT, created a minor stir in 2013 when she published her herbicide-celiac-connection findings. She argued that Roundup Ready's primary ingredient, glyphosate, may attach to the gliadin in wheat and help explain the explosion of celiac disease over the past fifteen years. "Glyphosate residues in wheat . . . are likely increasing recently due to the growing practice of crop dessication just prior to the harvest," she wrote in a paper she coauthored with Anthony Samsel in *Interdisciplinary Toxicology*. By her account the glyphosate finds its way into the kernels on nonorganic wheat and causes gut dysbiosis, or microbial imbalance. While Seneff and Samsel supported their argument with graphs showing a corresponding rise between Roundup use and celiac disease, I quickly point out that the mainstream scientific community does not back their conclusions; one researcher in the *Huffington Post* labels it "bad science." USDA plant geneticist Robert Graybosch told me, "I have actually never heard of anyone spraying Roundup just before harvest, and I recently read that only 5 percent of all wheat acres actually receive such applications." At the very least Seneff's assertion is worth a mention to indicate that in the absence of hard reliable data on celiac increase, speculative ideas abound.

One widely accepted theory, the "hygiene hypothesis," names cleanliness as a culprit. That term was coined by Dr. Erika von Mutius. When East and West Germany reunified in 1999, von Mutius, a health researcher, expected to find that children in the grimier, poorer Eastern Sector would be shown to suffer more from allergies and asthma than youngsters in cleaner, more sanitized West Germany. What she found, she reported, "was exactly the opposite."

Children in the polluted areas were less prone to allergies and asthma: exposed to more microbes early in life, she concluded, their immune systems developed more tolerance.

A comparative study of Finnish and Russian children living side by side on the border in the remote Karelia region bears that out. Now bisected, the area was once a single province, and the two populations are genetically related. As reported by *New York Times* journalist Moises Velasquez-Manoff in "Who's Got the Guts for Gluten," the wealthier Finns who practice good hygiene rank first in the world for type 1 autoimmune diabetes. For the poorer, less sanitary Russian Karelians, the disease is nearly six times less frequent, the risk of developing allergies one fourth as common. Living in a more sterile environment, the Finnish children are also five times more likely to develop celiac disease.

A Finnish scientist, Heikki Hyöty, suspects that the Russians' "microbial wealth"—abundant house dust and less filtered potable water—protects them from autoimmume disorders by strengthening their immune system, while the Finns' vulnerability can be ascribed to a decline in beneficial gut bacteria.

Health professionals I spoke to generally agreed that the hygiene hypothesis seems a credible factor in the rapid escalation, although several pointed out that the medical community, now much more alert to its symptoms, is also more likely to test for celiac disease than in the past and is therefore likely to find more instances of it.

Painful News from Down Under

If you think you're beginning to get a better grasp on the fundamental differences between celiac disease and gluten sensitivity, a word of caution: don't get too comfortable just yet. Fodmaps, those complex carbohydrates with unpronounceable names, have come along to further muddy the waters. Led by Peter Gibson, an Australian research team's well-designed study brought Fodmaps to the public's attention in 2013 as the probable cause of previously misdiagnosed non-celiac illnesses. This is where it gets interesting.

That same group at Monash University in Melbourne had previously presented the strongest evidence in a 2011 clinical study that non-celiac gluten sensitivity exists—so strong, in fact, that it made news around the world and gave a huge boost to theories about the prevalence of non-celiac gluten sensitivity, as well as to the GF market. In Gibson's double-blind study, neither the researchers nor the subjects, all of them complaining of intestinal distress, knew which wheat products contained gluten. Those who ate wheat with the protein experienced a return of pain, unlike most of the others. But in their new Fodmaps study findings, Gibson and team now refuted the earlier conclusion that non-celiac sensitivity was to blame.

Sorry, mates, they said in essence, we were dead wrong. Their new double-blind, placebo-controlled study tested thirty-seven individuals with gut issues who believed they suffered both from NCGS and irritable bowel syndrome (IBS). Gibson's team divided these subjects into groups with three different diets: high-gluten, low-gluten, and whey protein as the control diet. The subjects were put on a diet for two weeks in advance of the trial that contained very little if any of the Fodmaps group—fructose and lactose sugar molecules that in some of us produce gas, bloating, and fatigue, symptoms often misinterpreted as gluten-induced. Fodmaps are found in grains, milk, and at least forty-five vegetables and fruits including beets, squash, onions, sweet potatoes, eggplants, and sweet corn; apricots, apples, grapes, watermelon, mangoes, pears, and nectarines also make the list. If fermented only in the small intestine, they would be easily digestible, but Fodmaps also ferment in the large intestine, where they more commonly cause gastric distress. (Chiefly responsible is the fructan carbohydrate, containing sugar bonds we can't readily digest.)

Could Fodmaps in wheat, and not gluten, be the actual culprit? Gibson ran a series of diagnostic medical tests on the individuals as they spent a week eating from each of the three gluten categories. Keeping them off Fodmaps, he could accurately gauge the effects of gluten as an isolated ingredient. The researchers found that gluten on its own did not produce any changes in biomarkers or any intestinal inflammation, nor did it trigger an immunological response. In fact, the high-gluten dieters reported less fatigue and bloating than the other two groups.

The evidence led the team to conclude that Fodmaps in wheat most likely triggered those adverse reactions incorrectly ascribed to gluten. Gibson has revised his thoughts about gluten. He now believes that less than one half of 1 percent of us are victimized by non-celiac gluten sensitivity. *One half of 1 percent?*

That remarkable reversal raised my own curiosity enough to scout out Gibson and ask for a few more details. He turned out to be extremely generous with his time when we spoke by phone, and being an Aussie, affable and straight to the point. "Those books like *Wheat Belly* are very persuasive indeed, but the science in them is presented in such a way that it becomes pseudoscience because it is taken out of context and used inappropriately. An untrained person would not recognize that. Readers take their ideas as proof, which they're not. Our point of view, unlike theirs, is not evangelistic."

"Do you think people should stay away from wheat in any form?"

"Absolutely not! The Fodmaps fractions in wheat are prebiotic; they change the gut bacteria in a way that is believed to be quite positive."

Prebiotics, non-digestible fiber products, promote the growth of beneficial microorganisms in the intestines. Eliminating all Fodmaps for most of us is not a healthy diet, Gibson added emphatically. "The thing to do is to reduce them if you're having problems—cut out onions, for example, and see what happens. As for gluten, if you stop eating wheat or rye, you're giving up half your sources of fiber. You're inviting constipation. You won't do your gut bacteria any favors."

Perhaps the most noteworthy outcome of the 2013 follow-up was a discovery that went largely unreported: twenty of the thirty-seven subjects noted an increase in depressive feelings after eating gluten. "It may be that NCGS is more about things outside the gut; we don't yet know."

With no encouragement, Gibson voiced his impatience with the commercial exploitation of gluten-free in Australia as well as in the United States. "You don't know if advocates like Dr. Oz are doing this to promote their own products. There's so much money to be made. You start to worry about the advice that's coming your way. That's the academic view. It's my view, the one that still drives a lousy little car," he said with a laugh. "Any funds we're given go back into research." If you transform integrity and honesty into hard cash, in my view Gibson would be driving a Ferrari.

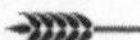

A large Italian study published in 2014 included 486 patients with suspected non-gluten sensitivity; they complained most frequently of bloating and abdominal pain, as well as headaches and foggy minds. Data was compiled from detailed questionnaires the patients filled out over twelve months at thirty-eight medical centers around Italy. "Based on our results, the prevalence of NCGS seems to be only slightly higher than that of celiac disease," the authors conclude. They put the actual figure at 1 percent of the population, slightly higher than the incidence of celiac disease and much more aligned to Gibson's extremely low estimate. Those are hard facts nobody appears to want to accept, not when 30 percent of us are cutting back or planning to cut back on gluten in the name of optimal health and slimmer waistlines.

Is it any wonder that the explosive popularity and staying power of the GF diet remains a baffling phenomenon to many, myself included. Are we suffering from a national epidemic of magical thinking, where hope pummels truth and blind faith overcomes reasonable doubt? To eminent food writer Michael Pollan, a witness to the fads and trends that have seduced us over several decades, it all makes perfect sense. "Americans," he writes, "are a notably unhealthy people obsessed by the idea of eating healthily."

Our long love affair with self-prescribed cures and restrictive diets began in earnest about two hundred years ago, and, wouldn't you know it, the food category that kicked off that first fad was grain, and the one grain that made all the difference was wheat.

The Cracker Man's Cult

The road to health is paved with good intestines!
—Dr. Sherry A. Rogers

When early American clergymen preached that cleanliness is next to godliness, they weren't just advocating a spotless kitchen or scrubbed feet as a path to heaven. They included the alimentary canal, that byway between mouth and anus. Alcohol was only one of many hazards to avoid. Another, according to some of the more extreme Bible-thumpers, was meat. It caused unclean thoughts—read sexual arousal—and led to self-inflicted bodily abuse—read masturbation. One of the leading proponents of that doctrine in the first half of the nineteenth century, Reverend Sylvester Graham, created a strict vegetarian diet centered on whole wheat as an antidote to, well, horniness. As you might guess, it was no fun. The wheat was compressed and rolled and baked into something hard and all but inedible, the first Graham crackers. No matter. For reasons that had nothing to do with getting rich off a gullible public, by the1830s Graham had launched the nation's first diet fad.

He was preaching his doctrine to a new breed of Americans. Touring the country at that time to research his classic *Democracy in*

America, the French aristocrat Alexis de Tocqueville observed us in those formative years to be obsessed with our own individual well-being. Sound familiar? De Tocqueville took that to be a by-product of something new and foreign to him, equality for one and all. "It is strange to see with what feverish ardor the Americans pursue their own welfare," he wrote, "and to see the vague dread that torments them lest they should not have chosen the shortest path that leads to it."

That could still stand as the branding strategy for every diet regimen ever devised to empty our pockets and fill our heads with fear that without it we might miss out on a better, thinner tomorrow. Graham may not have been a con man, but he was America's pioneer food cultist. He tapped directly into our insatiable yearning for self-betterment and cloaked it in religious sanctimony. Borrowing from matrimonial vows, the reverend preached that separating and removing bran during milling "put asunder what God has joined together." A purely intuitive, inspired guess on his part: biochemists would not confirm bran and wheat germ's storehouse of essential minerals or even formulate the concept of vitamins for another seventy-plus years.

Graham ingeniously connected the intestinal tract to the Higher Being. Coarse whole wheat, he argued, prevented "morbid action" in our bowels and under our bedsheets. Male masturbation was, he thundered, an express lane to damnation. A sure defense against that urge, brought about by the consumption of red meat, was a strict vegetarian diet abetted by the regular ingestion of the Graham cracker he invented. Maybe he was right. If you tried to eat one of Graham's original unsweetened, dense whole-wheat hardtack slabs, you couldn't possibly imagine anything as delicious as sex. He also advocated a host of other anti-erectiles like sleeping on hard floors and taking ice baths.

What Graham infused in his audience was a fundamental belief that a healthful diet laid the groundwork for a morally unimpeachable life. (He didn't live long enough to observe that Hitler was a vegetarian.) The reason we still remember him today is less for his questionable doctrine than for his marketing acumen. Fueled by fanaticism, driven by iron will, and powered by fiery zeal, he promoted his belief in religious purity via dinner menu to the yearning throngs, and they responded in vast numbers. Thousands of "Grahamites" crammed auditoriums along the East Coast whenever he lectured, and he toured tirelessly. More popular still were his essays and his 1837 *Treatise on Bread, and Bread-Making*. In that book he tells the story of a flour merchant who will not feed bread to his children at home. His daughter demands to know why. "Because, my child," he replies, "I know what it is made of." That was no gratuitous scare tactic: often chalk and even ground bones were smuggled into bread flour to bolster its white coloring. There were many rogues in the milling trade, and few enforced regulations. At the very least, Graham's whole-wheat bricks offered a safe alternative.

Perhaps inevitably the meat and wheat trade of the time, faced with declining sales, felt threatened and took umbrage—which in itself indicates the size of Graham's following. Outraged white-bread millers and bakers and butchers along the Atlantic Seaboard stormed his lectures in protest, to no avail: Graham's conflation of moral and physical health by then had reached a devoted audience of young males eager to pursue their own individual welfare, whatever the sacrifice. (Women, too, subscribed but in lesser numbers.) Some men lived in Graham boardinghouses that adhered to his strict eating regimen and restrictive practices; those dwellings also offered assurance to like-minded travelers that Graham's followers could find sanctuary on the road. A cholera epidemic in 1839 served to strengthen the reverend's hand. It created panic; there was no known cure or prevention. In that unhygienic era, Graham's creed of cleanliness, wholesome food, and abstinence appeased terrified and helpless urban dwellers.

In one form or another, genital or dietary, to Graham the culprit always came down to inflammation. Anything made from white flour or that once walked, crawled, or flew might inflame wanton desires. They represented an affront to God's handiwork on earth. Biblically correct wheat, whole and holy, fed the body, detumesced the loins, and placated the fretful mind. It became the sustaining victual of virtuous families, the mandatory staple for every meal.

What little I had previously known about Graham categorized him in my mind as yet another fire-and-brimstone historical health wing nut, the sort of fringe nutritional evangelist who draws large crowds, stirs up the rabble, incites riots, and ends up dying of the same disease his dietary scheme promises to prevent or cure. Not entirely inaccurate in this instance, but more to the point, when you put aside the religious dogma, the somewhat loopy insistence on ice baths, and sexual deprivation, also the ego-stroking fame that led him to make bolder and more outlandish claims as he packed houses up and down the East Coast, Graham had fastened onto a basic truth: whole foods make total healthy sense.

Four decades later another sexual abstinence advocate, Dr. John Harvey Kellogg, converted a Seventh Day Adventist sanitarium in Battle Creek Michigan into a world-class vegetarian wellness center for the rich and famous. Kellogg invented a flaked version of baked whole wheat—the first breakfast cereal. In time his ex–business partner and eternally feuding brother, Will, would figure out how to improve the process by using an easier medium, corn, on his way to creating an immensely popular breakfast cereal.

Grain cereals—there were over forty by 1900—began as health foods that had to be soaked overnight to be rendered digestible and barely edible. What Kellogg—vividly and wickedly portrayed in T. C. Boyle's novel, *The Road to Wellville*—and Graham shared, aside from egomania, was a repugnance of sex and a fundamental belief in the inseparable bond between spirituality, moral rectitude, and proper nourishment. Over time, however, the welfare of the stomach and the soul would part company.

Staff of Death

Many others after Graham came along to promote their own fit-body, fit-mind systems. At the turn of the twentieth century Horace Fletcher, a naturopathic physician, insisted that chewing each bite of anything you put in your mouth at least forty times—until it essentially liquefied—was the key to weight loss. Before long thousands were "Fletcherizing" their food. Moms and dad counted out loud and Jimmy and Janie chewed. Fletcher became a national medical celebrity on the order or Dr. Oz. The quest for self-improvement soon gave rise to the enormous popularity of fitness guru and muscleman Bernarr Macfadden, who often lectured dressed only in a leopard loincloth and tunic. White bread was one of his six pillars of sickness in America. In the first decades of the last century the handsome, buffed Macfadden launched America's first physical fitness magazine, *Physical Culture*, and soon built a mighty publishing empire. He started the Coney Island Polar Bear Club, whose members met at that playground to jump into the frigid Atlantic every winter. (They still do.) About white bread Macfadden had much to say.

He called it the "staff of death" and blamed it for his sickly childhood. In a chapter entitled "The White-Bread Curse" in his *Strength from Eating* (1901), Macfadden draws a few errant conclusions—"to use flour from which gluten has been removed is almost criminal," he writes because he considers gluten to be "the life-sustaining value in cereal foods." But his essential point was Sylvester Graham's as well: leaving out the bran and germ renders flour far more harmful than nutritious. To make his point, Macfadden reports on an experiment in which dogs fed entirely on white bread lived about as long as those given no food at all, while those fed on 100 percent whole-wheat bread thrived. "This proves beyond question that whoever is striving to subsist on white bread is starving a part of his body with almost as much certainty as if he were eating nothing at all, and that he will actually die about as soon as if fasting." He goes on to quote John Harvey Kellogg, who claims the hardiness of German peasants can be partly attributed to the black bread they eat.

Macfadden's flair for the melodramatic and tenuous grasp of factual accuracy may now bring a smile, but that pales in comparison with the influence he exerted on the public during his peak years. At the dawn of a new century he embodied a new and revolutionary approach to self-improvement through physical conditioning and proper exercise—his personal favorite being walking interspersed with headstands. What he and Graham both got right, of course, was that when all parts of a wheat kernel arrive in our digestive systems, they benefit us. And when they don't, they don't.

That brings up another topic: the sketchy relationship between purported truth, the basis of most food fads, and results drawn from reliable evidence. Graham and Macfadden, nut cases by some accounts but also keen observers with an intuitive intelligence, took a close look at the eating habits and general health of people in their day and age and noted a dismal state of undernourishment: at least about wheat, they guessed right. In the realm of food fads that does not often happen.

Many-Shaded Myths

The final verdict on gluten has yet to be announced in the court of public opinion, but as Michael Specter suggested in his *New Yorker* article, "Against the Grain," it might follow an arc similar to that of monosodium glutamate, or MSG, the ingredient in Asian (and other) food vilified since the late sixties as a cause of headaches and heart palpitations. Specter brings MSG to his reader's attention to make the point that "while there are no scientific data to demonstrate that millions of people have become allergic or intolerant to gluten (or to other wheat proteins), there is convincing and repeated evidence that dietary self-diagnoses are almost always wrong, particularly when the diagnosis extends to most of society."

As you might recall, the MSG scare began in 1968 with a letter to the *New England Journal of Medicine* pegging MSG—which pumps up the savory umami flavoring in food—as the cause of the letter writer's headaches and numbness. It quickly became known as the "Chinese-restaurant syndrome" and more or less overnight we declared ourselves MSG-phobic, seeking out clues to where it might be hiding in products while insisting to our waiter in Chinese restaurants that the cook not add a drop because we were highly allergic. Good luck to that. But in fact, as Specter makes clear, MSG is no threat; indeed it's identical to the glutamate ions our body manufactures. It exists naturally in tomatoes, mushrooms, and many other foods. Essentially we fell prey to a mythological food goblin—and that, of course, may well be happening yet again with gluten.

But food fads come in many shades, not always dark and foreboding. In the 1960s, America's leading manufacturer of wheat germ, Kretschmer, ramped up its ad campaign to target frustrated housewives and link nutrition to boudoir calisthenics. "Serve your husband this amazing food and see what happens!" ran the copy. Which they no doubt decoded as "Sprinkle a spoonful over his mac 'n cheese (he'll never know) and turn that bedraggled martini-sodden briefcase schlepper of yours into a stud muffin!"

In Kretschmer's print ads, frolicking married partners danced cheek to cheek or splashed together in the surf, prefiguring our current lascivious crow's-feet couples whose midlife foreplay heats up those spackled sunlight Viagra and Cialis commercials. For a time Kretschmer's bright red labeled bottles became a fixture in homes across America. Everyone over a certain age recalls Mom dousing Dad's and their corn flakes or Kix or maybe even the baked potato with that stuff, which tasted like embalmed sawdust. "It's good for your get-up-and-go," said Mom with a wink. Maybe, but as days became weeks, the half-filled bottle on the table rarely got up and went into anything we ate.

Which is the way of every food fad, it seems. In time an *e* floats past and attaches itself to the end of the word, and fads fade.

Winning Without Wheat

That may well be true for the gluten-free movement, but its demise at present is not in sight, which made me want to know more about its origin. I knew the trend piggybacked on the Atkins low-carb diet, but what provided its momentum?, I wondered. At length I came across Web and print scuttlebutt about a training experiment conducted by the 2008 Garmin-Transitions pro cycling team that competes in the Tour de France. Its inventive young sports physiologist, Allen Lim, I learned, listened to his riders' complaints about feeling bloated when carbo-loading on pasta before a race (during it they burn as many as 9,000 calories). When I tracked him down Lim told me, "It appears that for at least half the riders, they felt somewhat better when they eliminated wheat from their diet and substituted rice. But they needed to eat close to twice as much. Since then I've found that some athletes think it helps with their training and others think it's a ridiculous idea, it doesn't help whatsoever. Everybody responds differently based on their genetics. What we did didn't prove anything one way or another. But it did get people thinking about the issue. You can literally quadruple the amount of glycogen you store in your muscles and liver by increasing the percentage of carbohydrate, whether gluten's in it or not, and that's what is crucial. In a normal situation, you'd never do that, so it's all about context."

When Lim's balanced assessment made an appearance in *Men's Journal* in an article titled "Winning Without Wheat," it soon became a call to action—not really reflecting Lim's point of view. No matter. As Paul Simon sang, "a man hears what he wants to hear and disregards the rest." The news went viral. It carried a powerful message: if non-gluten works for professional athletes, it must be great for the rest of us, too. Health-conscious Gwyneth Paltrow soon became an ardent campaigner on her lifestyle blog, *Goop*. Other celebrities joined in and the anti-wheat movement took flight.

A Fad with Legs?

To gain a better sense of the staying power of the gluten-free obsession I contacted Harry Balzer, vice president at the market research company NPD Group, where he's tracked the food industry for more than thirty years. I expected Balzer to focus on GF's stupendous growth. Instead he focused on its marginal significance. "One in three of us say they want to cut back on gluten in their diet," he began, "but by 2016, gluten-free is projected to be only a $15 billion business."

"Only?"

"Steve, do you have any idea how big the food business is in this country? The amount of money we spend on food each year tops one trillion dollars. So that's a little more than 1 percent. Put another way, 99 percent of all the money spent on food in the country is not on gluten-free."

"Even so, it's everywhere. How come?"

"When probiotics hit with yogurt a couple of years ago, it opened up the door to marketing to anybody with digestive issues—and that's all of us sooner or later—so when gluten-free came along with the promise of processing wheat gluten without any problems, something that is supposed to be difficult to digest, true or not, it found a ready audience."

He compared it to the past popularity of the nutraceutical movement twenty years ago, and more recently the Atkins low-carb diet. "Gluten-free is just another novel way of saying, 'Maybe this is the answer to ultimate health.' We're always after something new and different. It's in our DNA."

Ideas or lifestyle changes that survive, Balzer continued, tend to do one of two things. They save money or they save time. "I haven't seen that with gluten-free, just a lot of people interested in it. At NPD we ask a thousand people every other week how they feel about certain issues. One is gluten, so I've been following this closely for about five years. The last two years it's taken off, and I'm not sure why except for increased publicity about the subject. That it hasn't crashed by now fascinates me."

"Is it a fad with legs, then?"

"If it only provides novelty, it's a fad. If it provides utility beyond novelty, it's a structural change, and that's more what this is, I think, a trend. But how long will it last? What people want now is low-cost protein, but when I look at gluten-free, I don't see an immediate return that you can measure, not time or money, so I think its future is limited."

"One last question, Harry. If $15 billion translates to, say, 1.5 percent of all food sales but 30 percent of the population claims they're cutting back or about to cut back on wheat and gluten, how come there's such a wide discrepancy?"

"It's the difference, Steve, between what you say you're going to do and what you do."

Bad Today, Good Tomorrow

Balzer's seasoned perspective got me thinking about the cyclical nature of our infatuation with the latest system-cleansing, fat-shedding, energy-boosting, brain-clearing, mood-lifting silver bullet—and the curious shifts of fate that befall the panaceas we pursue. For twenty years or more we marched in unison behind Nathan Pritikin and

Dean Ornish in their campaign against fat as the enemy of heart health and fitness. Now, in *Grain Brain*, Dr. David Perlmutter tells us, "Of all the lessons in this book, the one I hope you take seriously is . . . [that] fat is the preferred fuel of human metabolism and has been for all of human evolution." And where there's fat, there's potentially high cholesterol, which all of us know to be hazardous—or is it? Says Perlmutter, "Eating high cholesterol foods has no impact on our actual cholesterol levels, and the alleged correlation between higher cholesterol and higher cardiac risk is an absolute fallacy." As for eliminating carbohydrates, the basic Atkins diet and Perlmutter approach, Dr. Oz now warns that our brains depend on complex carbs as a fundamental source of cerebral energy.

These contrary decrees remind me that today's silver bullet may turn out to contain more lead than precious metal tomorrow, and the next day . . . well, that depends. Which is why, whether fad or trend, it's risky to predict the staying power of the gluten-free rush to judgment.

It's worth mentioning that the GF products cost an estimated 242 percent more that their gluten counterparts. What you get for your money is a modicum of assurance that you're not ingesting a protein with a rap sheet for causing digestive mischief. That comes at a high price to our intestinal tract and internal organs. The tapioca, corn, rice flour, potato starch, and xanthan gum, a polysaccharide thickener, most often used to create these alternatives lack insoluble fiber. As a consequence they metabolize so quickly that their glucose molecules shoot straight through our gut walls, promoting insulin resistance, obesity, and type 2 diabetes while adding little if any nutritive value. Judy Miller Jones and most other nutritionists also worry that packaged GF products reduce our intake of important vitamins and minerals such as iron, niacin, and riboflavin. You can avoid gluten without resorting to these products, of course. Pinterest and other Internet sites abound with sensible, healthful recipes that include quinoa and other beneficial, non-gluten wheat substitutes. The problem is, they're real food—and you have to cook them, not toss a frozen package of processed lasagna into your microwave.

Giving Up the Grain

To date I'd been observing the gluten-free landscape as if from an orbiting space station, that is, at a remote distance with nothing personal at stake. Thinking about it, that made no sense whatsoever for, as you might recall, the event that started me on this exploration was my wife's decision to stop eating gluten. After a month or more of listening to and reading about radical life changes brought about by eliminating the grain, I decided to hang up my rather tedious identity as a grizzled, skeptical journalist and try on a new mantle as adventurous experimenter. No wheat, no gluten for me, at least for a month.

"You'll be sneaking Triscuits at three in the morning," Bonnie predicted.

I expected to. I could hardly imagine not nibbling on a wheat cracker or—far worse—not sinking my molars into a chewy hunk of warm bread for that length of time. I tend to be both self-disciplined and masochistic—that is, I take a vow not to do something and I keep to my word, but in the end I usually wonder why I deprived myself.

The first few days of withdrawal reminded me of a silent meditation retreat I once attended. After arriving we crossed our legs, hunkered down on our zafu meditation cushions in a large, dimly lit room, closed our eyes, and, following our Zen master's instructions, began to pay attention to where each breath precisely entered and exited through the outer rim of our nostrils. Talk about fun! Twenty seconds into that exercise I was ready to bolt. No televised San Francisco Giants games for close to a week, no Pinot Noir, no cell phone, no music, no conversations, not a word to anyone. My monkey mind bounced hither and yon.

I somehow stuck out that first forty-five-minute meditation, and then the next, and slowly descended into a timeless space of self-reflection filled alternately with fear, yearning, wonder, and finally a submission to the unknown that was terrifying and joyful in ways I never expected. Five days later I floated out.

Dropping wheat from my diet, I can assure you, was far less profound and difficult, but it did follow a similar trajectory. It presented me with the unfamiliar and the uncomfortable, and challenged me to make peace with them. For four weeks or so I dropped the grain without substituting gluten-free alternatives—mostly things you serve to dinner guests you never want to see again. The sole exceptions were Mary's Gone Crackers, Kind granola products, and the quinoa pasta I traded for durum. I have a sweet tooth for salt, not sugar, so I wasn't sacrificing a craving for pies or pastries or other refined white-flour desserts and such.

Over the days that passed I listened with diminishing patience as well-intentioned friends encouraged me to pay special attention to the exhilarating changes I was soon to experience: increased energy, mental clarity, euphoric tranquility. Eventually I had to come to terms with the truth: I was a washout as a case study. Although I stayed with the program and didn't sneak in the occasional scone, those life-altering highs passed me by like leaves in the windstorm. When hungry, I noticed that I didn't anticipate with any real pleasure the thought of eating my next meal.

No steamy bowls of chewy al dente capellini pomodoro sat waiting to be inhaled and devoured in my fantasies. Food became boring. The primary takeaway was that wheat and I got along just fine, and that I missed it without craving it. But I still had no idea just how far off base wheat's adversaries were when they lumped white and whole wheat together as twin evils.

4

Slick Dough

> Tis a little wonderful . . . the strange multitude of little things necessary in the providing, producing, curing, dressing, making, and finishing this one article of bread.
>
> —Daniel Defoe in *Robinson Crusoe*

"Why is it," I'm asking, "that Cargill, ConAgra, Post Foods, or General Mills haven't mounted a kind of kick-ass defense of wheat—I mean with Super Bowl commercials and such? Not a word in public, not a peep. I get the impression, right or wrong, that you're running scared and hiding from the gluten-bashers. But wheat put you all on the map. General Mills boasted for years that their wheat flour 'makes the Bread of Life,' and I quote."

Brian Walker, technical service manager for Cargill affiliate Horizon Milling, a giant in the wheat industry, looks at me as if I just stepped off a steamer from a faraway corner of New Guinea. "That's usually not how things work in the retail sector," he replies with a gentle smile as if patting the family dog. "The usual practice is to come up with another product line that responds to the problem."

By which he means, by way of example, the three-hundred-plus non-gluten products that General Mills has added to its Chex, Pillsbury, and Betty Crocker lines—brownies, cookies, pizza dough, a huge assortment. The overwhelming use of processed white flour in these companies' products for close to a century might be primarily responsible for creating the problem they are now busy capitalizing on as a new revenue stream. Alternate wheat-free versions of classics like Bisquick shift the burden of responsibility to us as consumers to make the right choice, but that's asking a lot. "Our own physical body possesses a wisdom which we who inhabit the body lack," said the writer Henry Miller. "We give it orders which make no sense."

Not always, but when it comes to what we eat, the infant and adult in us seem to be locked in an eternal struggle for supremacy. Few foods of any sort appeal more to that insatiable child than sweet nothings and savory temptations made with refined white flour, fried or baked. Horizon is in business to mill it for mass-market wholesale bakeries like Grupo Bimbo. I'll be touring one of Bimbo's factories in Sacramento with Walker after lunch.

Both companies, like their counterparts everywhere, owe their existence to the invention of the roller mill, a breakthrough technology that replaced the millstones that had been grinding wheat into flour for at least eight thousand years. In the mid-nineteenth century, millers began to feed wheat kernels through a series of grooved metal cylinders spinning in pairs with slight gaps between them. The rollers split and scraped the wheat kernel without crushing it, as rotating stones do. That allows for a more efficient, complete separation of the starchy white interior, the endosperm, from the small embryo germ at the base of the seed and the fibrous bran that coats it. Clean endosperm, the source of white flour, seemed like a miracle of technology. For the first time lumpy flour with brittle shards of bran that could never be completely sifted off gave way to velvety, silken powder as white as snow. The roller-milled flour adapted to hundreds of uses, digested easily, and could safely be consumed without fearing a sudden molar-wrenching encounter with bits of hard fiber. Bakers could create cloud-soft pastries and breads from it, and, best of all, fluffy white flour could be made available for the first time at a price that the American public could afford.

The man who installed the first rollers in the United States about 150 years ago was an ex-governor and Civil War hero. In time his manufacturing company would scoop up competitors and rename itself General Mills. More about the mill owner—Cadwallader C. Washburn—and the origin of that revolutionary invention in a moment. At present Walker, facility manager Rich Rostomily, and I are seated at a small conference table at Horizon-Cargill Milling just outside Stockton. Cargill, which joint ventures with Horizon, is one of the world's largest producers and marketers of food and agricultural products; it buys, processes, and distributes grains and employs 167,000 people in sixty-seven countries. I was there to get a first-hand look at the progressive stages of industrial wheat as it moves from storage elevators in the Midwest to millers across the country to industrial bakeries to supermarkets, fast-food chains, and home kitchens.

Early on I'd been told that the story of wheat in America is a railroad tale. Beginning in the middle of the nineteenth century the grain's distribution from elevators, or silos, in Kansas, North Dakota, and elsewhere depended on lines like the Atchison, Topeka and Santa Fe Railway. As their fortunes ebbed and flowed, so, too, did wheat's. I was reminded of that connection when I arrived at Horizon earlier in the morning. Workers were unloading grain from a string of boxcars that sat on railroad tracks next to towering storage tanks.

"Rail is still the lifeblood of the industry," Walker tells me as we prepare for our tour. Based in the company's Minneapolis headquarters, he has experience over three decades in evaluating local market needs and delivering strategic guidance to key stakeholders from product management to wheat breeders to seed suppliers. He's also past chairman of the Wheat Quality Council.

Milling, during that time, has of course become ever more automated. By now I've become sufficiently familiar with its history, chronicled in a later chapter, to understand that we have ground and milled wheat kernels from the Neolithic era on to produce a white clean residue, the pulverized endosperm. The process never accomplished its goal to anyone's total satisfaction until steel rollers replaced stones. Since then, roller milling has dominated the grain industry.

The computers that now control every phase of the complex operation feed the raw grain kernels in measured quantities from those massive exterior cylindrical elevators beside the railroad tracks at Horizon, five stories high; they convey the kernels through conduits that transport them to the cleansing, tempering, roller milling, and sifting operations all required to transform hard small seeds, about one quarter inch long, into refined flour.

Tempering, as Walker and Rostomily explain when we start our tour, is the industry term for soaking the seeds in water for twelve or more hours. That toughens the bran skin so it holds together and does not powder, which would mix it in with the endosperm and darken the final product. Wetting eases the separation process.

For the next forty minutes as we tour the Horizon facility, I'm reminded that as engineering marvels, automated food processing plants like this one make a stunning impression. They perform complex mechanical feats in perfect lockstep. At Horizon conveyers glide tough-coated indigestible seeds through orchestrated stages of refinement without mishap within sealed walls to produce satin-smooth, fluffy endosperm. Unwanted parts of the kernel, the nutritious bran coat and germ embryo, get worked over by graduated rollers and various components until they finally break and sheer off to be sold as animal feed, while the white residue powder eventually gets bagged and transported to industrial baking facilities. From a health perspective, the entire operation may seem ass backward: the bran and germ should stay while the endosperm gets discarded. But there's no money in that, which is why only 5 percent of the nation's flour is milled whole.

Up close, surrounded by whirring engines cranked to high speeds, normal speech becomes impossible; you find yourself shouting to be heard by someone three feet away as if at sea during a howling gale. Hard hats and goggles are standard equipment. I can hear just well enough to take in what Walker is telling me, that the calibrated distance between each set of roller drums is progressively narrowed in every pass, or break, so that large bran-bonded protein chunks in the kernel's starchy interior are shaken loose and reduced to fine powder. That requires four separate runs; after each, an elevator lifts the milled kernels to the sifters on the top floor, which send particles down through gravitational shoots to the rollers for additional, finer pulverizing and separation.

"On weekends, one man at a control panel can run the whole automated operation," Rostomily tells me as we climb to the sifting room in a plant as big as a multistory office building.

About the top-floor sifter room: huge metal dumpster-style containers suspend down from the ceiling on wood rods that gyrate hundreds of times per minute, violently shaking the contents—split and scraped seeds—to loosen and discard the stubborn bran debris before sending the mesh-sifted contents down through those funnels for yet another looped passage between the steel rollers. "There's so much vibrating going on here," Rostomily shouts to me as the sifters vibrate so hard that the walkway trembles, "that people get seasick just standing where you are."

Later, back in the conference room, Walker tells me that when he got into the business, a few decades ago, 80 percent of Horizon's customers wanted bleached—chlorine dioxide–gassed—flour. Now it's more like 20 percent, except in the South, where the whitest of white flours is still in high demand. Every customer insists on a different level of enrichment, so that various quantities of nutrients in powder form are custom-injected with micro feeders back into the flour before shipping.

Enrichment, a subject I take up later, involves replacing a few of the many essential vitamins and minerals stripped out during the roller milling process.

"In a white-flour mill like this," I ask, "where do the bran and germ go?"

"Animal feed," Walker tells me.

"But they contain all the natural nutrients and fiber."

Walker nods.

"Which leads me to wonder, Brian and Rich, do either of you worry about eating the white flour you're producing, on a personal level? There's the gluten issue, of course, the sugar starch, too."

"We've been making and eating bread for thousands of years and doing just fine," Walker replies with a firm shake of his head. "I've been eating it all of my life and I'm perfectly healthy."

Rostomily nods in agreement.

"From a manufacturer's point of view, does the wheat backlash concern you?"

"Sure. We're down 15 to 20 pounds per capita, to about 135 pounds annually since the no-carb Atkins diet caught on. Of course the industry is concerned. Who wouldn't be? But what astonishes me is that obesity has been on the rise all this time we've been eating less wheat, so how can wheat be the culprit here? I don't get it."

I'm not quite through. "What exactly does 'bromated' mean?" I've often seen it on supermarket flour bags, more in the past."

"Potassium bromate is considered an oxidation ingredient," Walker explains. "One of the best and cheapest that was ever out there. It helps with oven spring, size, and volume."

"But it also causes cancer, I've read."

"In rats, yes, they found tumors. Based on tests done in Japan."

"Why isn't it banned, then?"

"It is in Japan and the European Union and Canada. The FDA encourages bakers to stop using it, but the agency doesn't prohibit bromate. In a few states like California, you have to label any products using it as carcinogenic, which, as you can guess, presents a marketing problem."

I can.

Baking Big

A few hours after leaving Stockton, decked out in white safety coveralls from head to foot, I am tipping my head to sniff freshly made dough in a large bin at Bimbo's wholesale bakery near Sacramento, which Horizon supplies. The headline copy on the Grupo Bimbo website reads: "Today, we are the most important Baking Company in the world on the basis of brand positioning, production volume and sales." From its humble origins in Mexico, Bimbo has grown to generate more than $13 billion in US sales alone; it also operates in Europe and Asia. I'd never heard of it before I began this project.

Sacramento's sprawling plant is one of more than a dozen spread coast to coast. By the time I make my visit I've been baking sourdoughs at home for a few months, and I've become familiar with the mildly tart, pleasantly winey scent emanating from my starters—bowls of the bubbling microbes that ignite the "sour" engine. The thick springy Bimbo soft-roll batter delivers a pungent kick I wasn't expecting, much more intensely vinegary than mine.

Surprisingly acrid and yet cloying, this all-white dough contains a heavy dose of commercial bread yeast, *Saccharomyces cerevisiae* (named for beer), a species that rapidly converts starch sugars to carbon dioxide and ethanol and produces the quick rise that wholesale bakeries seek. (The sourdough yeast, *S. exiguus*, propagates three or four times more slowly over twelve or more hours in a starter.)

Condensing that time span figures prominently into the battle plan of large commercial bakeries like Bimbo's, where all functions share one goal: to complete the baking process from fermentation to shipping dock in four hours or less. Before I arrive with Brian Walker, a guided rail system has already carried troughs of the thousand-pound leavening sponge, where the yeast is added, to a row of large metal bars that punch down that flour-yeast mass. The degassed dough is transported on conveyers to huge mixing bowls where sugar, dry milk, and as many as thirty "minor ingredients" are added.

By the time we show up about two hours later, the blended

dough has rested briefly in bins. During that interval, quick-acting yeast cells gobble up millions of complex carbs in the wheat starch and convert them to simple sugars. The final dough mix, now sitting in those bins, is about to start its second journey through the labyrinth of mechanical assistants designed to make and package it as fast-food hamburger buns. Rivers of leavened dough are positioned to slip down shoots into mobile trays of bun molds positioned on a roller-track system that looks to me like a miniaturized Disneyland ride. I am struck by the dual nature of the task this dough has to accomplish.

Food scientists have engineered its recipe to comply with Food and Drug Administration nutritional regulations, which account for some of the additives, yet the dough also needs to accommodate the demands of the equipment that will soon convert a thick slurry of water and powdered wheat into firm yet airy baked buns.

Water mixed with white flour of course is something that children use to cement pictures into scrapbooks. It's wheat or library paste. I remember the paintbrush my dad gave me in middle school to spread it all over a worn basketball when I cut up colored paper to make a globe of the seven continents for Miss ("Butterball") Key's geography class. I know all about its stickiness, too much in fact. I spent at least as much time cleaning up after a wheat-paste project as I did on the project itself. And when I stalled I paid a price: hard lumps of dried paste clung to the floor and table like barnacles.

Logic and personal experience tell me that wheat-paste glue is the last thing you want to try to slide down metal funnels as wet dough into those bun molds. It will never make it. It will stick to anything. Ah, but the Bimbo folks know that, too, as do all wholesale white-flour bakers, of course. Which is why they add chemicals and compounds like xylanase and hemicellulose in the UK to increase the dough's "tolerance to physical abuse during processing." In the United States, more vaguely, many of the chemical ingredients listed on the rear of a bread package "condition" dough for exactly that reason—to put it at the service of the machines that make it, not necessarily the health of the customers who eat it. That they can accomplish their mission without sickening us in the process is an impressive feat, but it does not mean they are contributing to our well-being. Slick dough contains biochemical equivalents of silicon lubricating oil. As a guide, I suggest scanning the rear label of your next sliced-bread loaf: the longer the list of ingredients, the less likely it is to be something unadulterated and highly nutritious to eat.

Fast and Furious

As I watch the batter-like dough drop smoothly into the mold trays, the Bimbo bakery foreman tells me with pride that his operation cranks out 150 bread loaves or 750 buns a minute. In the trade, any form of baked dough that transports food to your mouth is called a carrier—sandwich bread or, in this instance, buns.

"Seven hundred fifty a *minute*?" I may have misheard.

He nods. "And this is an older plant. You should see the new ones—they're turbocharged!"

Overhead bun trays whiz past in their mobile containers that dip and rise and skitter around corners on the winding track, shuttling the dough to preparation stations spread out to the far reaches of this capacious, single-story bakery. A heavy sweetness fills the air. At each stop robotic arms and automated equipment shape, bake, slice, bag, or pallet the buns for truck delivery to Bimbo's Northern California wholesale customers.

Speed, in this setting, dictates every activity. By reducing time on the bakery floor Bimbo reduces cost, satisfying a customer base that expects a low-priced product. Still, I've come to realize there is no mid-range price point for bread: there are artisan sourdough and other loaves at about $5 and up, or commercial bread at about $2 a loaf. Of course natural fermentation adds significantly higher cost, but still I wondered if Bimbo might be able to market long-fermented, more healthful sourdoughs available to the general public in the $3–$4 range without compromising quality. Fast fermentation, at the core of its strategy, speeds up the breakdown of starch sugars that feed the yeast. That translates to the rapid absorption of glucose in our bloodstream, and potentially to contributing to obesity, insulin resistance, and type 2 diabetes. Proteins in the gluten complex cannot be broken down into smaller, safer peptides unless naturally slow-fermented. This subject comes up again in much more detail when I delve into the benefits of sourdough processing later on, but it merits a brief mention here as one of the defining consequences of this common industrial approach.

Invited to peer in through the narrow window of a tunnel oven that stretches off into the horizon for what seemed like the length of a football field, I watch as countless ranks of white-dough buns in tight formation glide toward me on wide belts encircled by heating elements that transform their pallid tops into golden domes while delicately toasting their bottoms before tipping them into another set of mobile trays that will convey them to their next station. Row upon row the carriers march past, an impossibly long procession of identical browning globes.

Offered one, still warm, I'm jolted by a hit of doughy sweetness. If intended to mask the conditioners' chemical flavors, it does the job. The bun's soft, cake-like texture wavers between moist-air sponginess and balled-up facial tissue. With nothing substantial to bite into and in the absence of any definable grain taste, I forget what I'm eating in the process of chewing it.

But to fault the bun for lacking flavor and palate pleasure misses the point; designed to trap and hold moist, bulky ground meats and other weighty foods without collapsing into a soggy, dripping mess—that's why they are called carriers—these buns are meant to function as edible gloves, and in that they succeed.

Behind Closed Doors

How does a mammoth bakery balance industrial efficiency with nutritional integrity, I wanted to know. I was interested as well in whether Bimbo might be revising any of its bread formulas based on the current backlash against wheat.

If you are new to the name Grupo Bimbo, as I was, you'll more readily recognize some of its brands. In the United States they include Sara Lee, Arnold's, Brownberry Premium Breads, Entenmann's, Thomas' English Muffins, Oroweat, Freihofer's, Francisco, Stroehmann, the Ball Park buns I watched on the production line, as well as numerous other national and regional baked goods.

Founded by Lorenzo Servitje, whose family emigrated from Spain to Mexico City in the 1940s, the first single bakery dedicated itself to introducing American-style white wheat loaves to a population raised on corn tortillas. Servitje's son, Roberto, opened the company's first US bakery in Southern California in 1996. Going up against Interstate Bakeries Corporation and other major players across the US border, Bimbo flexed its muscles to scoop up competitors like Sara Lee. Along with the hamburger buns that make no claim to nutritional value, Bimbo, with US headquarters in Horsham, Pennsylvania, also produces Oroweat 100% Whole Wheat Bread and stresses its health benefits. *No high fructose corn syrup. No artificial colors or flavors. 22g whole grains per serving* reads the Oroweat label that emphasizes hearty flavor and fiber.

I also see calcium sulfate listed among Oroweat's ingredients. You might know the compound as plaster of Paris, included here to lubricate dough but more familiar to me as the rock-hard material used to make casts like the one I wore when I broke a thumb in college sports. In this context calcium sulfate, a "conditioning" additive, might be perfectly safe. To gain insight, I made an effort to contact Bimbo's Innovation and Nutrition Institute in Fort Worth, Texas, charged with developing and testing more nutritious, innovative products as part of its commitment to the World Health Organization. The institute is promoted on the company website as "one of the few of its kind in the U.S." Sending off an e-mail, I got back a two-sentence reply: "Thanks for your inquiry. That facility is no longer open." The Bimbo Research and Development group also blew off Brian Walker, who was trying to contact it on my behalf. General Mills also wasn't interested in discussing how it goes about the difficult business of balancing nutritional and commercial interests in changing times.

Fair enough, they have different priorities. One of mine is to trace the origins of roller milling; another is to chart the reward and cost of that invention.

5

Seeds of Change

All sorrows are less with bread.

—Miguel de Cervantes

The activity may go by various aliases, but it comes down to breaking and entering by force. When cereal grains—wheat, above all—reach maturity, we raid their vaults and loot their valuables, as we have for thousands of years, through a series of manual or mechanical scraping, shaking, and expelling techniques, all employed to penetrate the protective surrounding husk or hull in order to extract and consume the bounty within. Wheat adds its own complication by offering up an especially appealing and useful baking ingredient, endosperm. As the seed's white, powdery, tasteless, starch- and protein-laden major component, endosperm has always been the prize for bakers and consumers alike—a granular version of Aristotle's blank slate or tabula rasa.

This empty canvas awaits the brushstrokes of a master artisan or the swirling BeaterBlade attachment of a harried housewife dashing to get her cinnamon rolls or quick bread in the oven before picking up the kids from lacrosse practice. But of course, there's a catch: how to pry loose that soft, mealy interior while leaving behind undesirable, jaw-jarring seed fragments.

We solve that today with an elaborate rotating system of spinning steel cylinders and massive vibrating sifters. Three thousand or more years ago the Egyptians used rushes as sieves to separate out the larger chunks of shattered bran for regrinding, but they never succeeded in producing white wheat flour free from rock-hard fibrous shards. For as long as we ate wheat in some form up to the invention of the roller mill we paid a steep price, gnashing our teeth on those brittle bits and pieces buried within the white gold.

The earliest domesticated wild grasses, einkorn (*Triticum monococcum*) and emmer (*Triticum dicoccum*)—grown in Egypt—are both hulled, meaning that every two seeds sit inside an all but impenetrable fortress of tightly bound chaff, called a spikelet, that had to be soaked, dried, and fiercely thwacked just to free the seeds, which then had to be soaked and whacked again to separate out the edible meal from the husk or glume.

In a sense we hijack a wheat kernel—on average, there are about six hundred in every wheat plant—for our own purposes. As with all seeds, its intended design has nothing to do with us and has solely to do with the survival of the species. Each of the supportive components in any seed's germination has a specific role in nourishment or protection, and sometimes, as in wheat bran, both together. Over time we've developed shrewd methods of usurping those benefits by intercepting the life cycle for our own needs before the seed begins to develop. That intervention culminated with the nineteenth-century roller mill—breakthrough technology that, as soon noted, brought us our daily cheap bread and later left many health professionals wondering if we'd been too clever for our own good.

So closely was the plant—*Triticum aestivum*—identified with its starchy center that the name itself, wheat, is derived from the Old English word for "white," as in white flour. First cultivated at least ten thousand years ago, the earliest form of wheat played a key role in the Neolithic Revolution, our transition from migratory hunters and gatherers of food to sedentary cave potatoes who settled in one place and learned how to cultivate seeds and plants that entailed producing sustenance for the first time without the risk of being gored by an enraged woolly mammoth. A brief history of the plant's biological progression from then to today goes something like this:

Einkorn—not technically a direct ancestor of today's wheat but with the same forefather—began as a cross of wild grasses with two sets of seven chromosomes, a diploid. Soon after came emmer, a tetraploid (four sets) hybrid that resulted from human or natural crossbreeding, nobody knows for certain, and was first domesticated in Southern Turkey; Egyptians during Pharaonic times grew it along the Nile and extracted its softer, mealier endosperm to make flour—and by accident created the first leavened sourdough. Later the Italians adopted emmer and called it farro. This grain also gave rise to durum. Spelt, which came along a little later, about 5000 BCE, is a hexaploid, with six sets of chromosomes like modern bread wheat.

The takeaway according to anti-gluten proponents of einkorn and emmer (still available, see Appendix C and Chapter 11) is that they do not present that same health threat as contemporary wheats. (Even so, they still remain off-limit to anyone with celiac disease.) Grower and miller Jade Doyle at einkorn.com attributes the digestibility of ancient grains to three factors: that over time modern wheat has been crossed with two different goat grasses, introducing new less digestible proteins; that ancient grain's compact starches contain a higher ratio of slow-digesting amylose than amylopectin; and that ancient grains contain a much higher ratio of easier-to-digest soluble proteins to insoluble proteins than modern wheat.

To develop strains whose hulls did not adhere to seeds in order to expedite grinding and sifting, ancient planters must have experimented by trial and error. Somewhere, somehow they succeeded. It is these more genetically complex free-threshing varieties that have come down to us, tetraploid durum and the hexaploids with forty-two chromosomes in total. No longer does the hull bond with the seed, which eliminates a step in milling and much more quickly produces a larger quantity of flour. The wheat plant survived by becoming more utilitarian.

Here's what I find most interesting: *Triticum aestivum*, modern wheat, contains 164,000 to 334,000 genes, from eight to eleven times more than we do as humans, and is the largest genome of all agricultural crops. Wheat's genome today also contains about five times the amount of DNA as the human genome. (The genome includes all of the genetic material of a living thing, every instruction required for its creation and role.)

You can pummel me with these numbers until I'm woozy, I still find it hard to accept that the DNA in a spike of wheat outnumbers ours five to one. I grant you that humans are not an evolved species—we invented naked mud wrestling—but to be genetically humbled by a speck of grain, well, that still tweaks my self-esteem. As a member of the human race, I now seem to be slotted somewhere between a petunia and crabgrass.

Function over Flavor

Once free-threshing wheats replaced the first ancient varieties and offered easier access to the endosperm, cooking possibilities quickly expanded and functionality became the dominant theme. A ground-up version of the wheat plant's seed served so many food preparation agendas so well that a wheat variety's lack of any distinguishing personality or defining taste character evolved as an asset rather than a liability. Baking performance, as measured by gluten protein strength, took on much greater importance as centuries progressed. It gained so much leverage, in fact, that to this day strength rather than flavor or texture determines how wheat varieties are classified.

Strength may sound like a funny term to use to describe flour, which seems to have no substance or connective tissue whatsoever. Then, again, we're not cereal chemists. They define relative strength in wheat flour as the ratio of glutenin to gliadin. Simply put, it's a way of calculating the dough's ability to hold its shape without tearing (elasticity) and its ability to expand (extensibility). For most bakers, and for us consumers, higher protein flours make the most desirable breads. Numerous factors that determine strength come into play to tell commodity flour buyers in a few quick words what they need to know about the flour's protein content and baking potential. The nomenclature couldn't be more basic or simple: hard, soft; winter, spring; red, white.

Hard and soft refer to the texture of the grain during milling. Hard wheats shatter, soft wheats flatten out more like pancakes. Hard and soft wheats differ in protein levels. Hard wheats are grown in more arid environments, with lower yields and higher protein. The seeds of lower protein soft wheats fill more slowly in more humid environments, with more time to add starch. Industry has adapted to this, and now specs maintain the protein differences.

Unlike most other cereal grains, winter wheat, which accounts for 70 to 80 percent of US production, goes into the ground late fall or mid-spring. When sown before the ground freezes, the plants remain dormant during winter, then flower in spring and are ready to harvest usually in June or July. ("Flower" in a grasslike wheat produces no vividly colored petals, but mature spikes.) Spring wheat, planted from April through May depending on climatic conditions, is harvested in late summer or early fall. (Spring wheat can also be sown in fall in regions with a warmer winter, like California.) Most wheats are further classified by combining color, season, and strength, and so we get:

Hard Red Winter Wheat. Grown primarily in Kansas, Nebraska, and Oklahoma, it produces the amber waves of grain we salute in song as a tribute to America's limitless abundance and earthbound reverence for the bounty of nature. First imported as Turkey Red, named for its brownish red kernels, to the Great Plains by Mennonites emigrating from the Ukraine in the 1870s, hard wheat became the dominant wheat for much of the Great Plains bread basket a decade later with the introduction of the roller mill, the only efficient, fully functional method for separating out its endosperm. Though Turkey Red's kernels by comparison produced a small fraction of that starchy interior, the variety proved much more amenable to leavening due to the elasticity and extensibility of its abundant gluten. It succeeded because bread represents the bulk of most bakers' sales.

Hard reds range from 12 to 14 percent protein, the level required for optimal bread making. While higher-yielding cultivars eventually replaced Turkey Red, this class of wheat built Kansas. It still dominates the state's flowing fields, and as a class it accounts for at least half of the wheat grown in America and Canada. Kansas produces in the vicinity of 15 percent of the nation's wheat.

Soft Red Winter Wheat. Softer pastry-flour wheats come in at between 9 and 11 percent protein. The variety flourishes in more humid climates and is grown in Ohio, Illinois, and Indiana, as well as eastern Washington. Accounting for about 30 percent of the total crop, it is used primarily for pastry, crackers, cake, and breakfast foods.

Hard Red Spring Wheat. Another bread wheat—all breads are made from hard—its higher protein level can run to 14 percent, making it a valuable export to countries in Europe and Asia, which need to enhance their native soft-wheat blends. Adding up to about 20 percent of the nation's total harvest, it grows in our coldest states, North and South Dakota, Montana, and Minnesota, as well as in Canada, regions where winters are so severe that farmers wait until spring to plant.

White Winter and Spring Wheat. Both hard and soft, this wheat with a light tannish bran grows in the Pacific Northwest, also as a relative newcomer in midwestern states. It combines many favorable characteristics of bread and pastry wheats for pizza and home baking, yeast breads, cookies, noodles, and soft rolls. The hard versions are high in protein yet milder and sweeter than hard reds. Whole-wheat white flour might sound like an oxymoron, or simply moronic, but indeed you can use it to add the nutrition and fiber of whole-wheat flour to any baking project; don't let the lack of color confound you. To avoid confusion, visit the e-commerce website of the country's best national flour source, Vermont-based King Arthur Flour for a coherent explanation.

Durum. Spring wheat, the source for couscous and, of course, semolina pasta flour, grows primarily in North Dakota—the second-largest wheat-producing state. Yellowish durum is the hardest and densest of all wheats. It contains the highest percentage of protein, although not the kind that forms the strong elastic gluten bonds that leaven bread.

Making the Grade

There are few if any discernible varieties of industrial common wheat, a.k.a. bread wheat, that conform to the way we use the term to identify something by taste and texture—apples or wine grapes, for instance. There is no buzz about a delicious plummy Zinfandel blowing in fields of Nebraska or a creamy Chardonnay waiting to be threshed in Oklahoma. Names like Jagger, Overley, Fuller, and Postrock—leading Kansas wheat varieties—remain unfamiliar outside the heartland grain community. In fact, no distinctive flavor profiles exist among the many industrial varieties blanketing the Midwest from Canada to Mexico. (Durum might be the sole exception.) That absence of sensory traits shouldn't be confused, however, with an indifferent attitude toward quality. Another set of criteria comes into play.

Distinctions between one commodity wheat and another are called grades, as in Grade One, Grade Two, the top choices—and they matter much within the industry. Performance, not taste, dictates quality as well. Harvested bread wheat is graded on moisture content—too high, for instance, and it spoils when stored; also on dockage—the amount of extraneous materials like bits of straw or chaff that need to be sifted off before milling. The plumpness and integrity of the kernels are closely scrutinized, too. Shriveled, pinched, and damaged seeds reduce the crop's value. Nature sooner or later intervenes in the best-laid plans of growers, so gluten content has to meet a standardized percentage and is often adjusted in blending.

Grinding Labor

It's a fair guess that bakers knew a lot about the relative strength of various wheats long before anyone called gluten by name, and that preparing wheat taxed the strength of humans during its long reign as the planet's most widely planted crop. The true history of wheat's place on our table unfurls as a saga of perpetual human toil. Hand grinding both hulled and free-threshing kernels with primitive tools was miserable work, left (no surprise) to women and slaves. There were few things as arduous and tedious as stooping for hours over a saddle-shaped dish of seeds while pressing down a heavy stone rolling pin to crush them and extract their interior. During the Roman Empire the word for a bakery, or *pistrinum*, doubled as a common term for grunt work, chores nobody wanted to take on. Barley, more accessible, was also more fattening. (Gladiators ate barley, not wheat, to thicken up as a protective measure against minor cuts—so much barley porridge, in fact, that they were called *hordearii*, "barley men.") Samson was captured by the Philistines, who burned out his eyes. His ultimate humiliation in the biblical story is to be forced to grind grain in a Gaza mill.

Chewy all-wheat loaves high in gluten, *siligo*, were much in demand; slaves and soldiers ate dense barley bread, closer in taste to rye than wheat and made from dough with the consistency of clay. In later Roman times, by the first century silk was being used to shake fine milled wheat endosperm powder through the porous material while impeding fibrous matter. Imported from Egypt, Southern France, Algeria, and Sicily—wheat grows just about anywhere—grains were in time ground by querns. These first primitive "mechanical" grinders consisted of two circular stones, one stationary and the other mobile. They mashed wheat kernels between the revolving upper stone wheel and fixed bottom, smaller one while grain trickled down through a central hole; it was later stored in a hopper when the stones were mounted vertically. A thick horizontal pole connected the internal shaft to a blindfolded cattle or donkey, animals that trod in a rotational circle.

The hourglass-shaped Roman querns excavated at Pompeii, home to 33 bakeries at the time of its destruction in 79 CE, and elsewhere are much improved over earlier models. During Augustus's reign, a generation earlier, 250 Roman bakeries were producing about five hundred thousand loaves a day. By then Roman querns stored and fed grains into the grinder from above and were fitted with a socket between wheels. The rotating pole extended out through a portal from the central vertical shaft.

Constructed of two hollow cones, one inverted above the other, the exterior housing resembles a fantasy dwelling for gnomes in a child's fairy tale, but querns were no laughing matter to operate. Stone and clay versions traveled down through the ages at milling sites in the Mediterranean until Roman engineers were able to substitute surging water for animal power as the rotational engine. Wind in time became another option.

Eight miles north of Arles near the Rhône River in Provence adjacent to the Barbegal aqueduct, the Romans built one of the first massive water-powered wheat flour mills in the first century, "the greatest known concentration of mechanical power in the ancient world," according to one historian. Powered by Rhône River water channeled off the aqueduct into a sluice, two parallel sets of eight waterwheels turned sixteen grinding millstones, which produced an estimated 4.5 tons of flour a day. The overshot waterwheels were constructed one above the other on a steep hillside, so that the run-off from the higher wheel drove the one below it, and so on down the line.

What remains today at Barbegal, spread over the length of a football field, is a kind of ancient mill blueprint made up of piles of stones that delineate a descending staircase bordering a series of collapsed walls once housing the waterwheels and grindstones. The Barbegal mill's bread fed the entire population of the region, thought to be between ten thousand and thirty thousand inhabitants, while the aqueduct itself supplied all of the area's water.

Pliny, Cato, and others report that reeds and linens and numerous mesh fabrics took on the role of sieves employed to trap inedible seed coat and germ fragments deposited by the crushed kernels. Until roller mills and mechanical sieves joined company, pure white flour required arduous human labor as well and proceeded more slowly than grinding.

Bones of Contention

The cheap dark "peasant" bread of the masses also contained white flour, but in a much smaller ratio to the brown and tooth-crunching bran and oily germ that came along for the ride. So pervasive was the association between dark bread and impoverished laborers among Romans, Greeks, and others that to gauge a person's social status, you simply noted the hue of her bread and, most likely, the condition of her teeth.

H. E. Jacob, author of *Six Thousand Years of Bread*, an eccentric and entertaining compendium of fact, factoid, and lore written by a man who survived a Nazi concentration camp by baking loaves out of sawdust, insists men and women had been white-flour crazy forever, and that the elite in every society prided itself on the lack of color in its bread as an index of noble breeding. Jacob quotes a fourth-century BCE cookbook author, Archestratus, who told of Greek gods sending Hermes to Lesbos to buy some of the island's whitest-of-white flour for them. "In order of merit, bread made from refined flour comes first," wrote Diphilis, a Greek dramatist from the same period. "After that bread from ordinary wheat, and then the unbolted wheat made from flour that has not been sifted."

Some bakers and millers added non-grain ingredients—ground-up bones, alum, mashed cooked potatoes, chalk, and even lead—to whiten their bread. Tobias Smollett, in his picaresque comic novel, *The Expedition of Humphrey Clinker*, wrote in 1771 that "the good people are not ignorant of this adulteration" that turns bread into a "deleterious paste" but are willing to sacrifice their taste and their health because they prefer it to wholesome food, and "the miller and the baker is obliged to poison them and their families, in order to live by his profession."

Dental excavations dating back six thousand years to Egypt, where leavened bread was first discovered, indicate that Egyptians all too frequently bit down on something so indigestible, it might as well have been a pebble or glass shard, but it was in fact a fibrous seed skin, small enough to avoid detection yet sharp enough to cause painful damage. Even the highborn suffered; despite the unlimited supply of slave flour-sifters at his disposal, the teeth of Pharaoh Amenhotep III (1391–1353 BCE) were discovered to be worn down to the nub by chewing wheat. Thirty thousand workers who built the Great Pyramid of Cheops at Giza were paid daily in bread, not money, at three loaves a day. It was a currency that came at a high cost to creature comfort.

That could explain why there haven't been more pyramids. As stone-milling techniques improved over the next two millennia, they produced finer, more desirable grain flour. Still, limitations in the materials and design ruled out the near-total separation of prized white from brackish brown bran and germ in large quantity at reasonable cost. That came about only with the invention of the roller, which was brought about by a toothache.

White Gold

The whiter your bread, the sooner you're dead.

—R. P. L. Clark

In 1830 in Switzerland an engineer known to history simply as Müller went to a dentist and altered the future path of bread and wheat. A discussion with the dentist about whether teeth would actually be necessary in the future, based on the turn in early nineteenth-century Europe toward soft foods, sent Müller home with thoughts about the difference between crumbling and crushing a grain of wheat. In that era, millstones chewed up wheat kernels and pulverized them in a "low grinding" action that, like molars, shattered hard surfaces in a single pass and deposited all three parts of the original grain in the flour. But, posited Müller, what if a nonchewing mechanism, like toothless gums rubbing together, compressed the seed until it burst and spit out the naked endosperm, leaving behind the unwanted materials.

That principle of separation by compression (and scraping) led to the construction of the first roller mill in Switzerland, which promptly failed. Engineer Jacob Sulzberger soon came along to redesign the corrugated iron rollers so that each, spinning in an opposite direction, was independently steam-driven. That tweak worked so efficiently that the mill became a highly profitable success. With additional sifting, historically expensive white flour could be produced in quantity and made available for the first time to an average consumer at an affordable price.

While softer varieties dominated much of Europe, harder, higher-protein wheats, which did not respond well to millstone grinding, blanketed Hungary and would eventually find their way from Russia to America. Hungarian millers out of necessity quickly adopted the roller as a much more efficient alternative. They experimented with porcelain and iron cylinders, both of which gave way to grooved steel, stronger and more durable. The new invention spun, compressed, and spit out the starchy interior into a lumpy substance called middlings, which was then hand-sifted and reground. By the time Americans began to pay serious attention to this invention and ultimately pilfered its design, Hungary had mastered the subtleties of mechanical flour milling.

Pirated Bounty

Enter Cadwallader C. Washburn. His name may seem better suited to a marquee of a W. C. Fields comedy, but his shrewd business acumen and ambition cast him as the John D. Rockefeller of wheat processing. The flour company he founded in Minneapolis eventually acquired several competitors and changed its name to General Mills. A Civil War hero and soon afterward elected governor of Wisconsin, Washburn realized early on that if you capture the water power rights to a river's surging falls, you then buy up all the land at the foot of that falls and lease it to prospective mill owners at a sizeable profit.

Whether they planned to mill wool, cotton, or lumber, in his pre-electricity era it mattered not: they all needed the fall's hydraulics to run their machines, as did Washburn and partners, who built a series of stone-ground flour mills on that same land starting in 1866 and the massive centerpiece Washburn "A" mill in 1874. When it blew up in a spectacular flour dust explosion and fire caused by poor ventilation in 1878, killing fourteen, a new mill was erected but not immediately equipped.

Rumors by then had been circulating that millers in Budapest were discarding millstones in favor of steel rollers. The Hungarian enterprise was shrouded in secrecy; in Great Britain, the adoption of rollers introduced by Henry Simon, who developed a system with a vibrating sieve, was still in its infancy. Traveling to Hungary to learn more, Washburn contacted the milling engineer responsible for designing the cylindrical roller mills and commissioned him and a Bavarian engineer to do the same for an experimental wing of Washburn's rebuilt factory.

When these men faltered, Washburn replaced them with a Frenchman, William de la Barre, who went back to Hungary, talked his way into a new roller mill as a night worker, made surreptitious sketches of the machinery, and then fled to Vienna with his diagrams. Arriving back in Minneapolis, he presented visual and written notes sufficiently detailed to pirate the design and begin manufacture.

Rotating at different speeds, the two rollers perform complementary functions: the slower roller holds the kernel, and the faster one strips off or shaves its germ after the first break. Seeds pass through a series of break rollers that separate out fine particles, the white flour; most of the cracked seed remains middling—a combination of endosperm, bran, and germ particles. That coarse mix undergoes multiple passes through reduction rollers and sieves until cleaned of all but a small percentage of bran and germ.

For the hard-hulled bread wheats that were now being planted and grown in the Great Plains, rollers proved up to the task, and that mattered: stone milling never achieved similar results. The roller technique was so efficient that when I visited Horizon 150 years later, in 2013, I encountered a twenty-first-century version of the same basic engineering design, now abetted by computerized purifiers and sifters.

End of an Era

Once the industry established that roller mills did a superior job at less expense and produced a flour with much more popular appeal, they rapidly replaced the nation's small, picturesque gristmills, scattered over the wheat states to serve local farming communities. One author, looking back from the vantage point of 1925, lamented the passing of those quaint, rustic stone-ground operations with their overshot waterwheels. He recalled them as "the favorite of the poet and the writer of fiction from time immemorial." If the old mill survived, he added, it did so "only as a ruin." With it went the iconic miller, often the most powerful (envied, feared, loathed, respected, despised) figure in the village, depending on how honestly and efficiently he carried out his stone-ground craft.

There are really no precedents for the revolutionary impact of roller milling in the long history of any grain. The closest comparison might be cotton; Eli Whitney's invention of the gin transformed a stubbornly uncooperative fiber that had resisted mass production into a cash cow, as did roller milling for wheat. It gave us what we wanted, the prized white fluffy gold, in a quantity we could only dream about until then. A few earlier inventions led to it: the automated stone mill, put into use by Oliver Evans, and a more recent one, the purifier, which harnessed compressed air to blow off the bran from ground middling grain.

There would soon be nothing local or bucolic about milling. Viewed through the prism of processing, wheat's closest relatives were now ore, gravel, and plastic, materials whose value fluctuated in proportion to how well they responded to roller reduction. A crop that would be engraved on the back of a copper penny and imbedded in our collective mythology as a symbol of America's rural roots and unlimited natural resources became a commodity. Charting our course to an industrial society, wheat gave birth to agribusiness behemoths like ConAgra, Cargill, General Mills, and Pillsbury.

Trouble in Paradise

Roller mills provided us with the nation's first processed food—a boon to one and all, it appeared. Slightly sweetened, uniformly white sandwich slices with spongy, cake-like consistency pleased everyone in the house. The kids did not have to be threatened or bribed to eat it. The bread stayed fresh more than a day, sopped up gravy, and fed the family at an affordable price. (Breakfast cereals, by contrast, emerged from a fitness-inspired whole-grain movement and for years connoted good health at the expense of good fun—until 1939, with the introduction of the first sweetened cereal, Ranger Joe Popped Wheat Honnies, which became an instant success.)

But there was trouble brewing in paradise. Within a decade after rollers replaced millstones, some American and British doctors reported a rise in coronary heart disease, diabetes, and gastrointestinal problems that they suspected were linked to the popularity of the refined carbohydrates in white flour. One physician, Charles Edward Shelly, wrote to the *British Medical Journal* in 1924 that with the introduction of roller milling, "a vital injury was inflicted on our national well-being . . . [the flour] lacks the proteins, fats, vitamins, and mineral constituents present in the original grain, providing only an emasculated substitute which is not merely inefficient, but also directly harmful." Few initially paid much attention. In France and England, as Michael Pollan and others point out, a growing number of medical practitioners, Shelly among them, noted that "Western diseases" occurred less frequently in Asian and African countries; the British medical teams who served the colonial empire there kept accurate records. A sharp rise in chronic illness rates followed the introduction of white flour and sugar.

The widening recognition of refined flour's deficiencies—no mystery to Bernarr Macfadden and body fitness advocates as far back as 1900—prompted an American chemist, Benjamin R. Jacobs, in the 1920s to investigate the loss of essential minerals in white bread. They included B vitamins thiamin, riboflavin, folic acid, and niacin, as well as iron. Two B-vitamin-deficiency diseases, beriberi and pellagra, became much more common across America, as did anemia. The first head of the FDA, Dr. Harvey Wiley, wanted a law passed to ban the use of bleached refined flour, while Jacobs called for manufacturers to add back essential nutrients. Congress—it will come as no surprise—did nothing for another two decades.

Running on Empty

Endosperm is a source of quick but short-duration energy, the Oreo cookies your mom added to your backpack that gave you a sugar spike. It occupies the vast bulk of the wheat kernel, about 80 percent by weight. Our saliva contains the enzyme amylase, which begins to help digest its starchy carbs as soon as we bite down on them. We're partial to pastries that, we say, practically melt in our mouth because that in fact is what they do: the flour immediately begins to degrade in response to the enzymatic interaction between two complex carbohydrates in the endosperm, amylose and amylopectin, and our saliva's amylase.

The bran (15 percent by weight) and germ (5 percent), meanwhile, house almost all of the seed's vitamins and minerals. Once removed, they were—and still are at Horizon's Stockton plant and elsewhere—sold off to feed livestock.

While the government and bread companies did nothing to improve the nutritional value of processed wheat through the Depression, war accomplished what common sense and a capitalist economy failed to do. As we prepared to send our first troops off to fight in World War II, physicians and health professionals looked closely at the eating habits of raw recruits. Draft board doctors and dentists rejected half of the first million men screened for active duty. These unfit young Americans, they discovered, consumed more calories from white wheat bread than any other source. America's would-be fighting forces were eating spongy air, essentially running on empty.

To improve their conditioning, in 1942 the US Army announced that going forward it would purchase only enriched flour. In time, content analysis would confirm that refined, unenriched white flour delivers only 20 percent of the seed's twenty-two vitamins and minerals, half of its calcium, and a scant amount of its fiber. It delivers none of the germ's essential fatty acid (omega-3) or linoleic acid. The fibrous bran contains about 70 percent of the seed's pyridoxine (vitamin B_6), 85 percent of the niacin (B_3), and more than 70 percent of its phosphorous, potassium, zinc, magnesium, thiamin, and manganese, as well as the majority of its pantothenic acid (B_5), copper, and calcium. The germ accounts for all of the seed's vitamin E, and the bulk of its thiamin (B_1) and folic acid. B vitamins improve appetite, vision, skin health, digestion, cognitive and nerve functions, and protein efficiency, as a partial overview of their function.

If your eyes slide off the page while browsing numbers, as mine do, consider this image provided by grain historian Ted Hazen: "I knew someone who worked in a big merchant flour mill in Buffalo, New York. One time I asked him what do they do to control rats and mice. He answered, 'Nothing! We let them eat all of the white flour that they want, and we find them with their little stomachs blotted out, dead of malnutrition.'" Until rollers replaced stones, millers everywhere were plagued by insect infestation in the grain. "They vanished 'cause they ain't stupid," one said. "There's nothing in the white for them to feed off."

Vitamin Shots

As we entered World War II, the War Food Administration, now only too aware of the damage done by not regulating the bread industry, made an all-out effort to bolster all retail white flour with vitamins and minerals. At symposiums around the country, bakers learned to inject milk solids and vitamins into their dough. Bread, they strategized, was the one food product consumed by poor and rich alike, the most widespread vehicle for toning up our citizens. Congress passed a law requiring compliance in 1943. To enrich white flour, bakers replenished it with iron and four B vitamins. (If calcium is also added, the bread is "fortified.") General Mills teamed with the chemical manufacturer Merck to speed up the process, but many Americans, most of whom still know nothing about vitamins, were wary.

Many housewives equated enrichment with richness, as in things that make us fat. Major propaganda efforts ensued. One slogan, "You're in the Army, too!," caught on as a pitch to make buying enriched bread a patriotic duty. Once the war ended, the law was repealed, but many states enacted their own mandates. Today, thirty-six states follow FDA safe standards of enrichment.

While that process addresses none of the health issues related to white flour's role in quickly elevating blood sugar—and thereby increasing the risk of diabetes by overworking the pancreas to produce insulin, higher cholesterol levels, and a welter of related conditions—it did lower the rate of ailments caused by B-vitamin deficiency. By 1950 pellagra death rates dropped in the South from 10.5 per 100,000 people to 0.5, a tenfold decrease. In 1998, the FDA added folic acid to prevent some birth defects, according to the Mayo Clinic, and lower the risk of heart disease.

Still, enriched flour is missing large quantities of at least fifteen minerals and vitamins available in 100 percent whole wheat. It delivers an average of 34 percent of the B vitamins, 30 percent of the minerals, and 21 percent of the fiber, while adding more riboflavin (429 percent) and iron.

How much benefit from these artificial vitamins and mineral compounds are we actually receiving? They come from external sources, not from the kernel itself. That prompts some biochemists to bring up the Humpty Dumpty syndrome, as in: once you pulverize a wheat kernel and extract its carbohydrates, you rupture the seed's internal synergy among bran, germ, and endosperm, and degrade the kernel's nutritive value. No artificial replenishment strategies, they say, provide an adequate substitute for the nutrients in their natural state.

Professor Joanne Slavin at the University of Minnesota Department of Food Science and Nutrition focuses on food intake and its effects on intestinal microflora. Her advice: substitute whole for refined grains across the board; don't just add whole grains to your diet.

At the Children's Hospital Oakland Research Institute (CHORI), staff scientist David Killilea compares commercial flours to determine their mineral content. Breaking open kernels, he explained, exposes them to oxidation. "You change the internal chemistry, just like swirling a glass of wine. Roller milling oxidizes wheat more than stone grinding; it strips off nutrients and fats like lecithin that are part of the plant's own immune system."

When I visited his lab, he showed me his equipment. A spectrometer allows him to detect the presence and level of specific minerals, each emitting its own color. Killilea uses his equipment to determine if there are adequate amounts of basic minerals in standard all-purpose flours like Gold Medal. "You need minerals like magnesium, which are way below adequate levels," he said. "Those are easier to put back than complex vitamins, which the heat of roller-milling damages. Once you add in oxidation, they're all but impossible to replace, like the seed's vitamin E. More that 90 percent of us don't get enough in our daily diet. Enrichment doesn't pick up the slack."

Fellow CHORI microbiologist Dr. Mark Shigenaga compares white refined flour to alcohol in its disruption of the intestinal wall. It produces, he says, its own version of a hangover. "The foods that make us want to take a nap after we eat are the ones to avoid."

Many, if not most, contain pulverized endosperm. "Its job is not there to feed us," Killilea reminded me. "The starch in that wheat seed acts as baby food to feed the baby plant, which needs a huge carb source and amino acids as it develops. It also needs nutrients. They don't come from the endosperm. They come from the aleurone layer and germ. We've co-opted this plant by tossing out those nutrients to obtain all-purpose flour with a long shelf life."

There's more, of course. There's the aleurone layer Killilea mentioned, a protein tissue that wraps around the endosperm and delivers phytochemicals, vitamins, and minerals to us in whole wheat but does not survive the refinement process. In addition to keeping the fetus healthy in pregnant women, the high level of folate in the aleurone layer plays a major role in preventing cervical cancer. It is also the most proficient producer of antioxidants; it, too, gets lost in processing.

And finally there's phytic acid. Seeds store phosphorous in that form as an energy source for the sprouting and germinating plant. In the Paleo diet it is considered an antinutrient (something that blocks a nutrient) because it binds minerals such as iron and zinc and inhibits their absorption by our bodies. We cannot take advantage of phosphorous for ourselves in wheat—it strengthens teeth and bones, among multiple benefits—unless we get an assist from nature to penetrate the phytic acid bond and trigger its components to become accessible.

Nature obliges with a microbial aide that goes by the name of phytase, an enzyme whose job it is to release bound minerals during germination. For us, Killilea explained, long fermentation over eight or more hours allows enzymatic activity to unlock the phosphorous as it loosens the bond, making its contents bioavailable.

Short fermentation, vital to the speedy four-hour start-to-finish process at wholesale bakeries like Bimbo's, does not allow sufficient time for that to happen, he added.

Killilea's detailed grasp of the plant's survival stratagem once again got me thinking about the astonishing way that nature goes about its daily business of reseeding the world we live in on its own cyclical schedule, not ours. As a microbial scientist, he viewed wheat as a natural resource we've exploited in order to make it commercially appealing and easily digestible, at some cost to our intestinal equilibrium. His concern was educating consumers, not condemning the industry.

"A happy gut," Killilea reminded me as I left his office, "is the key to health."

Inside the Hull

That trade-off between good and good-for-you was becoming a recurrent theme as I made my way into the heart of wheat. That reverse strategy, I thought to myself, adds a second meaning to "refined" beyond smoothly textured. The flour is well mannered, too, glad to be of use and eager not to offend. Year-to-year performance consistency matters most, and few would dispute that the approach has a legitimate place in food preparation. At the same time, it does no justice to the grain's potential as an enticing and enriching source of pronounced taste discoveries—a void now being filled by the local artisan wheat movement, which is dedicated to introducing consumers to organic, heritage wheat varieties that are both wholesome and full-flavored.

I wonder if commodity wheat hasn't become too amorphous for its own good. We know that those finely milled particles quickly flood our bloodstream with converted starch sugars. As I was about to learn, brutal climate conditions have combined with consumer resistance in the wake of the non-gluten, low-carb trend to lower industrial wheat's appeal both to farmers and to average American families, if for different reasons. It's always been tough to make a buck growing wheat, farmers say, and it's not getting any easier, so perhaps the time has come for Big Agra to take a long look at producing wheat varieties that do more than spring up as white and bland as cloud puffs in Betty Crocker's oven.

Whether that happens or not, it won't have any immediate effect on a crop now in trouble, and one with a noble past: I discovered modern wheat to be the grain that half a century ago played a heroic role on the world stage, when a breeder named Norman Borlaug created a wheat variety that saved millions from impending starvation.

7

Survival of the Shortest

> Food is the moral right of all who are born into this world.
>
> —Norman Borlaug

In the summer of 2014, for wheat farmers and breeders in the Great Plains, issues raised by the gluten-free backlash ranked as the last thing on anyone's mind. Survival was first and foremost. A prolonged drought and a dwindling market presented challenges that eclipsed all other considerations. The decline in the grain's popularity since 2000 reflects public interest in lowering carbohydrate consumption, says the USDA. You wouldn't know that by charting shares in Krispy Kreme's doughnuts, which have soared 800 percent since 2009, but even so there has been a steady slippage, and worse news ahead as studies continue to connect high carb intake to a range of maladies.

As other crops attract former wheat growers, less wheat is being planted. Corn and soybeans, buoyed by strong export demand, fetch a better price per bushel for less effort, and drought tolerance of both crops has been improved. By 2012, corn plantings exceeded the acreage dedicated to wheat almost two to one, ninety-seven million acres to fifty-five million acres. Nebraska farmers now plant and harvest only one half the wheat they once did. In 2014, due to stress created by the lack of rainfall, growers harvested about twenty bushels an acre, while in a year with adequate rain they bring in forty bushels on average.

US commodity wheat, the wheat you and I eat in packaged bread and boxed cereal, no longer occupies its lofty position as America's iconic food crop. Those severe weather extremes brought about almost certainly by climate change spotlight its vulnerability. Last year, in the midst of a brutal Grain Belt drought, Kansas reported its worst wheat crop since 1989. Mary Knapp, service climatologist in the Department of Agronomy at Kansas State University, gave a shrewd assessment of the situation: "You can have a drought punctuated by a flood and still be in a drought," she said. "If the rain comes too quickly, it doesn't have a beneficial component." All Grain Belt crops suffered, but wheat got hit the hardest.

It takes about as long to recover from a drought, Knapp added, as it did to reach drought status, so if it has been three years in the making, it will take three years or more to recover from the effects.

From one point of view, that's farming; that's you battling and befriending nature, or vice versa. That's what you sign up for when you choose not to sit in a cubicle and sneak a peak at World of Warcraft while allegedly tracking how much gross revenue fell to the bottom line in last month's sales report. You might learn as a grower over time to make peace with or resign yourself to nature's capricious and potentially destructive behavior, but shifts in popular food consumption trends, added to agricultural volatility, can knock you sideways.

Wheat growers in Nebraska, as elsewhere, have on both accounts hit a rough patch, and they don't garner a whole lot of compassion. When a few of them pulled into a gas station diner in the western part of the state with USDA research geneticist Robert Graybosch one day last summer, another farmer, a stranger, approached them.

"Why are you boys so dirty?" he asked, noting their mud-caked clothing.

"We've been out in the fields."

"Doing what?"

"Checking out our wheat."

"*Wheat?*" the farmer snorted. "You can't do *nothin'* with wheat!"

In six words he summed up a prevailing Grain Belt consensus: the time and resources put into growing wheat today doesn't pencil out compared to corn, the cheap fructose source for carbonated sodas, along with crops like sorghum and soybeans. Burdened with its weed- and pest-control and irrigation issues, not to mention its meager profit margin, you're most likely backing a lame pony.

For industrial wheat farmers the number-one driver is yield. After that come consistency and baking performance. All three are now in jeopardy.

Modern Menace?

I sought out Bob Graybosch on two separate occasions for a different reason but took full advantage of his intimate knowledge of Nebraskan wheat to gain insight into the current status of the crop. As a plant geneticist, Graybosch, a transplanted Long Island native now located at the University of Nebraska at Lincoln, knows what goes on inside the chromosomes of a wheat plant. That aroused my interest because plant genetics are at the crux of the anti-gluten argument, which, as presented by William Davis, Mark Hyman, and others, goes something like this:

While there is no genetically modified wheat, the grain we eat today is the result of crossbreeding efforts over the past sixty years, which have resulted in alterations that in modern wheat shorten stems and enlarge heads. Let me pause the conversation for a moment to clear up a common confusion about breeding methods. Genetic modification, or GM, introduces the gene of an entirely unrelated species into the DNA of a plant. An example would be DNA from bacteria immune to Roundup herbicide inserted into wheat to produce a Roundup Ready seed. That wheat seed would grow into a plant genetically altered to survive intact when Roundup is sprayed on or around it to kill weeds.

There is no GM, or transgenic wheat. No external species like Roundup bacteria have been inserted into the gene pool. Selective crossbreeding within the species has produced all of the alterations. Using that method, Davis and his proponents argue, wheat breeders have tampered with modern wheat's gluten proteins. As a consequence the wheat we now grow and eat in America bears little or no resemblance to earlier versions, heritage and ancient strains like einkorn and emmer. According to the Davis camp, the gluten molecule itself has mutated to produce a more dangerous version of one its proteins, gliadin.

To strengthen his argument in *Wheat Belly*, Davis cites a 2010 paper in *Theoretical and Applied Genetics* that tells us that "modern wheat breeding might have led to an increased exposure to CD [celiac disease] epitopes." An epitope is part of a molecule, an antigen, perceived as foreign and attacked by the immune system. But he neglects to add the paper's next two sentences: "On the other hand, some modern varieties . . . have relatively low contents of both epitopes. Such selected lines may serve as a start to breed wheat for the introduction of 'low CD toxic' as a new breeding trait." In plain English, the researchers are telling us that crossbreeding is hard to track for such changes, if any, in the makeup of gluten, and that there is no conclusive evidence either way.

In the *Huffington Post*, Dr. Mark Hyman writes, "We eat dwarf wheat, the product of genetic manipulation and hybridization that created short, stubby, hardy, high-yielding wheat plants with much higher amounts of starch and gluten and many more chromosomes coding for all sorts of new odd proteins. The man who engineered this modern wheat won the Nobel Prize—it promised to feed millions of starving around the world. Well, it has, and it has made them fat and sick."

That man, Norman Borlaug, saved more human beings from death by starvation than anyone in history—no exaggeration, and I'll get to him soon enough. But first, if these broadsides against "modern wheat" with shorter stems and larger heads ring true, the Green Revolution hybrid developed by Borlaug, wheat most of us eat today, has to be considered a modern menace. If true, the plant's mutations gave rise to a steady increase in celiac disease since the mid-'60s and are directly responsible for gluten sensitivity. Were we still consuming the same wheat as our ancestors, the argument goes, wheat would not be thickening our waistlines as it destroys gut walls, stiffens joints, shorts out neural synapses, and betrays our minds and bodies in ways large and small.

I suspected that once past the attention-seeking hyperbole and hysteria, there might indeed be a legitimate case to be made about a damaging increase in mutated gluten in Borlaug's dwarf wheat, which is why I contacted Graybosch, an expert in the field.

He initially replied in an e-mail, "The assertion that wheat breeding has changed the amino acid sequences is probably without merit." When we first spoke a few days later, he told me that his university department did a comprehensive study for *Crop Science* in the early nineties on older and modern dwarf wheats using sophisticated technology to determine if indeed Borlaug's wheats were higher in gliadin and glutenin, gluten's two components, as Davis would some years later claim.

They weren't. "We compared, for instance, a semi-dwarf called Karl 92 with Cheyenne, selected from Turkey, one of the original wheats grown in Nebraska in the 1800s. There was no difference in their relative proportion of gliadin."

"So I'm not eating more gluten in my bread today than in the past?"

"Only it's added by the baker. In the plant it hasn't changed at all. In fact, we could actually be consuming less gluten than great-grandpa did. It's actually been remarkable that protein levels have been kept sufficient enough to satisfy the demands and specifications of the industry."

The typical Nebraska wheat head is no bigger than that of Turkey, Graybosch continued, and the ratio of gluten to starch remains constant. Numerous other plant geneticists I spoke with draw a similar conclusion. Graybosch told me that when he came to the University of Nebraska in 1987 he looked at wheat quality—not a measurement of its nutritional value, but of its baking performance.

"Strong doughs are at a premium; they have to stand up to a lot of physical abuse." I was reminded of my experience at the Bimbo bakery. But strength does not equate with an increase in the percent of gluten, which has held steady at 12 percent on average, he told me, for more than a century.

I ran the same questions about a possible upswing in modern wheat's gluten proteins past Brett Carver at Oklahoma State University. A wheat breeder and chairman of the National Wheat Improvement Committee, Carver talks with a honeyed drawl that most actors in Southern roles strive to imitate without coming close. Borlaug, he said, was interested in increasing yield. "It's like swimming upstream to try and improve yield *and* to improve protein content." They work against each other. "Scientifically there's no way of increasing the gluten content in modern wheat when you're crossbreeding for yield."

Carver, like numerous plant geneticists I talked with, was only too ready to unload on William Davis and, in Carver's view, his fellow fact-fudging wheat-bashers. "They concentrate on gliadin, which is a crazy attack, because gliadin is *not* the main show. It's glutenin. If breeders changed any protein, it would have been glutenin, there's so much more of it. And they didn't."

Both Carver and Graybosch make the same point about Borlaug's genetic target—a single gene controlling the height of the plant. "When you have a gene that is responsible for one trait that resides in a different chromosome from another trait—in this case, height and gluten richness—they don't tend to be co-inherited. Whatever Dr. Borlaug accomplished has no effect on an increase in gliadin. That's where this argument really breaks down."

"Now that we know the wheat genome," Graybosch adds, "we can see that the dwarfing genes are not on the same chromosome arms as the proteins."

"But Borlaug couldn't take advantage of any of this mapping."

"Oh, no, he was flying blind."

Stan Cox, senior plant breeder at the Land Institute in Salina, Kansas, and an author of several books including *Sick Planet: Corporate Food and Medicine*, told me that "Davis shows a complete misunderstanding of wheat breeding," as did the dean of gluten researchers, Donald Kasarda, now semiretired and in his early eighties. Kasarda put forty years into studying and characterizing gluten proteins. If it fogged his mind, I saw no sign of that when I visited him in his office at the Western Regional Research Center in Albany, California. "I think there could very well be something called wheat sensitivity," he speculated, "but if true, I think these people are responding to something other than gluten. Nobody really knows."

Taking note of the current controversy, Kasarda decided to broadcast his own findings. In the *Journal of Agricultural and Food Chemistry* in 2013 he published a detailed genetic history of wheat with elaborate charts and graphs that track gluten levels in the United States for the past hundred years. Kasarda show them to be consistent, no higher now than they were at the start of the twentieth century, still between 12 and 14 percent, and not in any way mutated into a "new," more dangerous form. Based on his reputation as a respected agricultural scientist and the *Journal*'s high standing as a publisher of peer-reviewed studies, Kasarda's paper quickly became the go-to reference to refute "super gluten" theories.

"One reason that celiac disease has increased sharply may be that we're eating more gluten in the concentrated form of vital gluten. It's in everything," he told me. "It's highly processed, and a lot of products contain vital gluten, that pure gluten concentrate used to boost low-protein bread doughs and bind ingredients. But there's *not* more gluten in the dwarf wheat itself." Kasarda takes deliberate misstatements about wheat gluten as a personal insult. His voice rises, his neck muscles tighten. Tamper with the truth as he knows it from a lifetime's work and you are apt to catch a knuckle sandwich.

The debate will continue, but for the moment my money's on the geneticists. The evidence that modern wheat contains more gluten or more "odd new proteins" than in the past or that gliadin has become more pernicious seems unsubstantiated by hard evidence; it doesn't hold up to rigorous scientific scrutiny.

What does pass muster is Borlaug's extraordinary achievement.

Falling Stalks

You quickly grasp the problem that breeder Norman Borlaug was trying to solve if you picture the body of an elephant attempting to walk on the spindly legs of a whooping crane. Wherever wheat grew on more than six hundred million acres around the globe, from the Arctic Circle to the equator, from high in the Himalayas to the rim of the Black Sea, the swelling heads of tall wheat plants, rising four feet or sometimes much higher, sat on wobbly, hollow straw stalks. As these heads grew heavier with maturity and absorbed moisture, the weak straw below often bent or collapsed, and row upon row of toppled plants simply rotted in the fields. For eons this process, called lodging, plagued wheat growers. It became more ruinous still as farmers increased nitrogen applications, called inputs, in the twentieth century to enlarge heads and boost yield. Combines, those giant farm machines that reap, thresh, and winnow grain, cannot efficiently retrieve lodged wheat, and no one had come along with a workable solution.

Norman Borlaug, the greatest world savior I'd never heard about, took on the challenge. His lab was a scorching Mexican wheat field. His original equipment included a dilapidated wooden plow that he strapped to himself, like an ox, then pulled on foot to till the soil when he first arrived at Ciudad Obregón in the Yaqui Valley region of the Mexican state of Sonora in 1944 under the auspices of the Rockefeller Foundation. Trained as a plant pathologist, he was charged with developing crosses (hybrids) that resisted rust, a rampant, ubiquitous stem fungus that infects wheat plants, breaks stems, kills leaves, and shrivels seeds. Rust causes serious epidemics in wheat-growing areas all around the globe. When Borlaug arrived it had demolished much of Mexico's modest wheat crop.

Borlaug set about to plant seeds and cross the resulting varieties until, by evolutionary laws that govern the survival of the fittest, he could select out wheats that did not succumb; crossbreeding thousands of them, over several years he eventually arrived at reliably fungus-free lines whose kernels he then germinated in large volume to produce healthy seeds for Mexico's farmers. Normally, as Washington State University plant geneticist Steve Lyon explained to me, a breeder needs ten years to develop a new variety that can be planted with assurance. But Borlaug was faced with a crisis—not the last—and responded to it by setting up two breeding stations, one in fall and one in spring. In practice, that meant planting thousands of mongrel wheats to create four that showed good rust resistance. Local farmers at first wanted nothing to do with him.

"For a while," Borlaug later recalled, "hardly any of them would even talk to me." Still, when his crosses proved rust-resistant, word spread, farmers planted, and in time he was able to corral several dozen talented young scientists from various countries, including

India, to join him in Mexico, where he acquired the detailed knowledge he put to use about fifteen years later to breed a wheat variety with a single gene mutation that overcame the threat of mass starvation.

To meet that crisis and provide an inexpensive, lifesaving source of daily calories and proteins where most needed, in impoverished countries, he realized his options as a wheat breeder were limited: he could not redesign or reinforce the long, hollow straw that failed to hold up the vertical head. But what if he could shorten and maybe even thicken it, so that it became less of a flimsy branch and more of a trunk? Given the lack of sophisticated analytical lab equipment available to him, Borlaug had set himself an all but impossible task. One gene might make the difference, but which gene among the hundreds of thousands, and how to locate it?

If the stakes were not so high—life-and-death for millions—Borlaug might have bailed. But by the mid-'60s it had become only too clear that we'd managed to breed ourselves faster than we could feed ourselves. The planet had run out of arable land. Population growth continued to exceed food supply at a rate that would create widespread famine by the 1970s and devastate large areas of Africa and Asia. India's population every year was now increasing 5 percent more than its agricultural output. The words of Thomas Malthus, who predicted in 1798 that "premature death must in some shape or other visit the human race," echoed down through time, and there was a recent precedent.

As the Great Leap Forward in China (1958 to 1961) unraveled, an estimated forty-five million Chinese died in the worst of all twentieth-century famines—a result of Mao Tse-tung's catastrophic decision to outlaw private farms and establish agricultural collectives. Poorly equipped and chaotically administered, they failed to harvest enough wheat and rice to feed the population. Coercion, terror, and violence followed; the country's moral code collapsed. Some resorted to cannibalism. Mao's response: "When there is not enough to eat, people starve to death. It is better to let half of the people die so that the other half can eat their fill."

Converting vast swaths of pristine wilderness areas to farm acreage might avert the immediate calamity, but future generations would be forced to pay a disastrous environmental toll for our inability to achieve a sustainable balance between agricultural production and population growth. Political leaders were essentially helpless. An international delegation approached Borlaug, by then known as a visionary innovator within his agricultural community, a man with the single focus, imagination, talent, and skills of the very few who change the way we live. And Borlaug knew his history. While wheat is not in reality the staff of life—on its own the grain lacks lysine, one of the nine essential amino acids required as building blocks for new proteins—it figures prominently in our physical and spiritual evolution: wheat acted as an internal engine for the expansion of Western civilization and in wafer form to this day it symbolizes the body of Christ. There are thirty-eight verses on wheat in the New Testament alone. Because of its abundance and reliability as a source of protein and calories, more than any other single food, including rice, wheat has come down to us time and again as representing a last defense against mass starvation.

Seeds of Hope

Earlier in his facility at Ciudad Obregón, Borlaug had experimented with the seeds of a cross between a short Japanese wheat called

Norin 10 and another line, Brevor, sent to him years before by a gifted breeder, Orville Vogel, from Washington State University. They failed at first to perform. Borlaug ascribed that to the seeds, but in fact it was human error—his own. Until he planted the seeds under favorable conditions—artificially hibernated (vernalized) in a cooler to simulate a winter wheat—he had no success.

Finally, when they sprouted in a second attempt years later, he decided to cross that winter dwarf to produce a spring variety for planting in warm countries. Earlier efforts had produced unappetizing bread. To combat impending world famine, he became obsessed with the idea of producing a dwarf wheat whose short stalk would not bend or collapse under the weight of a heavy head and whose kernels contained sufficient gluten protein to make an acceptable loaf. He also had the idea of creating in that same cross a wheat that would produce not one but two crops a year in different temperate zones.

His next step was to execute his concept. Bear with me while I walk you briefly through the minutiae of crossbreeding. Nothing better demonstrates Norman Borlaug's willingness to take on the most laborious, painstaking tasks in difficult surroundings—a boiling-hot Mexican wheat field—with tenacity and persistence.

Wheat seeds or kernels, as you'll recall, grow inside protective, ladderlike, fibrous, self-pollinating spikes that send out needle shoots or bristles, called awns. Each spike contains an interior floret, which houses three green nubs, or male anthers. As the plant matures, the anthers will contribute to creating new seeds. Your first job in crossbreeding is to emasculate—that is, castrate—the florets by cutting off their tops and dislodging the anthers.

With tweezers or forceps in one hand, a scissors in the other, and a broad-rimmed hat to protect against blazing sun rays, you separate the sleeve folds that enwrap them—each anther is about the size of a slender match head—then very carefully and gently, with those forceps, pull them out, more or less like removing an embedded splinter. A single spike may contain as many as fifty florets. From experience in a wheat field I can vouch that this endeavor requires a keen eye and way more patience than I will ever possess. You're performing agonizing plant surgery at close to a microscopic level as sweat blurs your vision and lubricates the fingers you're trying to use for a firm grip. Leave just one anther behind accidentally and you can easily sabotage the entire enterprise. As one plant breeder remarked, "It doesn't take much in the way of brains to sit on a stool in the sun for hours and pollinate a few hundred plants, but it sure does take a cool hand."

Only the female pistil should remain intact. You then cover the emasculated spike with a glassine bag, and do the same with the intact spike of the second plant you want to mate it with.

Part Two of the backbreaking, shoulder-cramping procedure involves rubbing the emasculated florets with an anther from the second plant a few days later, then gently joining them together side by side and covering the pair with a bag—a granular version of bridal night. In time, if you're successful, the new cross seeds that develop in the emasculated florets through cross-pollination will carry the genes of both plants.

Now, imagine performing that tedious procedure 8,156 times—Borlaug kept track—until, with no guidance provided by genome mapping, you at last arrive at the cross you've been seeking, the one-gene mutant that delivers high yields, pest resistance, and good bread, and flourishes in two contrasting temperature zones. (Previous efforts sometimes met two of the three, but not all requirements.) From that effort of over several years of exhaustive work, he finally isolated four fully functional seed varieties.

Their most striking feature was that they no longer resembled traditional four-foot wheat. His cross, called dwarf (and sometime later, semi-dwarf), stands only about two feet high on a stocky stem, within reach of a combine's reaper, with larger heads for greater yields. "The seeds in these four packets," writes one of Borlaug's biographers, "represented his greatest masterpieces. They could open horizons higher and wider than any known."

As they did: today, over 90 percent of all the wheat grown around the world is a dwarf variety. Borlaug then "blew it out"—that is, germinated seeds from thousands of his dwarf crosses as quickly as possible in two locations—one at sea level in the Yaqui Valley, another high in the mountains at seven thousand feet in the region of Toluca. That "shuttle breeding" experiment, invented by Borlaug, enabled farmers to grow two successive plantings within the same year. Conventional wheat breeders who worried about subjecting new gene crosses to radically disparate conditions considered his revolutionary approach dangerous and foolish.

He proved them wrong. By 1963, only a few years from the first planting of dwarf spring wheat, Mexico's yield increased threefold, and Borlaug's new variety comprised 95 percent of it. Mexico, for Borlaug, was an ideal agricultural lab. If he could grow vigorous disease-resistant wheats in a country with such limited resources, he could transfer what he had learned to other struggling nations. By the early 1960s he had apostles in nine countries including M. S. Swaminathan, now head botanist at India's leading agricultural research center.

Before Borlaug performed his breeding breakthrough, mass starvation still seemed inevitable. "I have yet to meet anyone familiar with the situation who thinks India will be self-sufficient in food by 1971," biologist Paul Ehrlich declared. And for good measure: "India couldn't possibly feed two hundred million more people by 1980." Ehrlich famously wrote in his best-selling book, *The Population Bomb*, in 1968 that "the battle to feed all of humanity is over. In the 1970s and 1980s hundreds of millions . . . will starve to death in spite of any crash programs embarked upon now." America could not and should not save India, he argued, because "the world has too many people." Ehrlich called it an epiphany.

Growing up in a village in India at that time, Kulvinder Gill told NPR's Dan Charles "it was a common belief that this world is going to end because of starvation. People are going to fight for food and kill each other." For Borlaug it was a call to action.

He arrived in India and Pakistan in 1963 and began testing his new varieties of Mexican dwarf wheat, the seeds of the Green Revolution. Economist Walter Falcon, deputy director of the Center on Food Security and the Environment at Stanford's School of Earth Sciences, was with Borlaug in South Asia. "A character and a half, that was Norman," Falcon recalls. "He worked for thirty years and stressed his wheats in every possible way to come up with robust varieties that could hold their own against pest and climate and disease problems." His greatest contribution, Falcon adds, was to cross and cross until he got the same results in winter and spring wheats. "What he and his team did was phenomenal. He couldn't understand when any of us asked about how he expected to finance the work. He took it as an insult."

A relentless array of maddening obstacles gathered like squalls at sea to capsize Borlaug's efforts. Mostly they took the form of "bureaucratic chaos, resistance from local seed breeders, and centuries of farmers' customs, habits and superstitions," he'd later write. "One of the greatest threats to mankind today is that the world may be choked by an explosively pervading but well camouflaged bureaucracy."

By all accounts, Borlaug rarely lost his temper, and in a career that required him to challenge entrenched attitudes wherever he traveled, that equanimity helped win the day. In India he managed to convince the political powers to change national policies to release his new seeds and provide the large amounts of nitrogen-based fertilizer needed for wheat cultivation.

Falcon remembers Borlaug as being driven and fearless. "He brought in fifteen or so tons of seeds to India that he somehow got past all the inspection agencies and organized their planting. Almost never do you want to do that, plant without testing first, but here there was a crisis and Norman didn't flinch."

His numerous critics warned that no single improvement in wheat's genetics could stave off the catastrophe about to befall millions in Asia and Africa. He called their overly cautious approach "scaremongering" and set out on his own path.

After the first Indian crop proved successful, Borlaug managed to bring in 250 tons of dwarf seeds in 1965, the year war broke out between India and Pakistan. He sent 350 tons to that country as well. Fortunately, as a result of emergency wartime regulations, the grain monopolies in both countries lost their power to block the distribution of his wheat. "If it hadn't been for the war, I might never have been given true freedom to test these ideas," he'd later remark. In 1966 the Indian government purchased 18,000 tons.

Farmers who planted his seeds soon confirmed their superiority; within a few years India's wheat production increased exponentially. The maximum wheat yield from hand-harvested small scattered plots amounted to 800 pounds per acre in 1963; by 1968, Borlaug's varieties increased that yield to 6,000 pounds per acre. Against great odds, almost to the point of spinning the globe backward on its axis, mass starvation never materialized; one wheat gene mutation prevented it, and there have been no famines in India since then. During those decades the country has become self-sufficient in food. So, too, has Pakistan. It progressed from harvesting 3.4 tons of wheat in 1966 to 24 million tons in 2014. India's wheat production has increased from 11 million to 95 million in the past half-century; in both countries grain production has outstripped population growth.

At about the same time, in 1966, the Rockefeller Foundation, a crucial ally from the start, agreed to help fund CIMMYT, a Spanish acronym for the International Maize and Wheat Improvement Center, in Mexico, and to install Borlaug as director of its wheat program. Employing advanced technical equipment in the field and lab under Borlaug's direction, the center, headquartered near Mexico City, established one of the world's largest free seed banks. To date the nonprofit has distributed 158,000 wheat varieties around the globe to researchers and impoverished farmers and now employs more that seven hundred people in thirty-eight countries. It counts more than ten thousand researchers as alumni.

Writing in *The Atlantic* about thirty years after the first dwarf seeds were sown, Gregg Easterbrook would look back over Borlaug's achievements and single him out as "the man who saved more human lives than any other person who has ever lived." (That line, uncredited, found its way into just about every Borlaug obituary.) Although in the United States the geneticist's name still remains largely unknown to the general public, Europe and Asia took notice early on. When Borlaug's wife, Margaret, went looking for him on a hot afternoon in 1970 in Obregón to let him know that he had just been awarded Sweden's Nobel Prize, she found him knee-deep in a field of wheat.

He thought someone was playing a hoax on him. No agricultural scientist had ever won the prize. His Nobel citation praised him for "turning pessimism into optimism in our dramatic race between the population explosion and the production of food." A Presidential Medal of Freedom and Congressional Gold Medal followed, along with dozens of other accolades that included the American science community's highest award.

Not a man who dwelled on past accomplishments, Borlaug kept his eye on things to come, and he didn't like what he perceived. "I am deeply concerned that we are taking mankind to the brink of disaster in hopes that a scientific miracle will save the day," he told a meeting of the World Bank.

When he died at ninety-three in 2009, Borlaug had lived to see his innovations in crossbreeding produce immense increases in yield where most needed. In his last decades, however, Borlaug also witnessed a furious backlash. As we use the term *green* today, the Green Revolution he is famous for originating is anything but. It's now dependent on inorganic petrochemical inputs in the field, most crucially nitrogen fertilizer, as well as lab-created herbicides and pesticides. The large-scale monoculture farming of dwarf wheat occupies all but a small fraction of America's fifty-five million acres.

For Borlaug, a Texas A&M professor in later life, if keeping billions alive through chemistry entailed supplying inorganic fertilizers like ammonium nitrate to India and other endangered countries in the mid-'60s to grow dwarf wheat (and rice, piggybacking on his techniques), so be it: without that high-yield nitrogen boost, wheat plants would have delivered shriveled seeds and thousands, if not millions, would have perished from starvation.

No enemy of healthful living, to Borlaug organic farming methods were admirable but not adequate to the task. "There are six billion people in the world. The organic movement at best could feed only four billion. I don't see two billion people volunteering to disappear," he said. Close to twenty-five thousand people around the world still die from hunger every day, he pointed out. "If these [organic advocates] lived just one month amid the misery of the developing world, as I have for sixty years, they'd be crying out for tractors and fertilizer and irrigation canals and be outraged that fashionable elitists back home were trying to deny them these things."

By the 1980s those environmental-group "elitists" were applying enough pressure on nonprofits like the Rockefeller Foundation to impel them to back away from funding high-yield agriculture in sub-Saharan Africa thirty years ago. A decade later, former president Jimmy Carter was finally able to intervene on behalf of high-yield dwarf wheat in Ethiopia, which recorded a 32 percent increase in production the following year. Still, today in Africa subsistence wheat farmers lag far behind their counterparts in Asia.

In battles waged on this front there are no triumphant victors and one inevitable victim, common sense, at least by Borlaug's reckoning. If clearing more arable land requires millions of acres of deforestation, he argued, and if high-yield genetics provides more food on less acreage, then reducing the demand for new farmland pays off in saving our woodlands and wilderness from destruction.

That line of reasoning became known as the Borlaug hypothesis, and it seems to hold up to close inspection. Cereal production today has doubled or more in many areas of Asia while cultivated lands have increased by only 4 percent. But having dueled with crusading activists and lobbyists for many decades by the mid-'80s, he held out little hope that his environmental opponents would ever revise their thinking based on factual evidence, no matter how persuasive.

Nor is that likely to deter anti-glutenites like Mark Hyman who, as you'll recall, insists that Borlaug's efforts did nothing more than "make people fat and sick."

It served as a reminder that no good deed—or great deed, in Borlaug's case—goes unpunished or gets acknowledged by narrow-focused advocates who cannot see beyond their own agendas.

Frankenseeds or Not?

A final word about GM, since it looms like an ominous shadow over any discussion of wheat breeding. Borlaug was a proponent. So, too, are many of the industrial wheat growers I spoke with. They note that at present 90 percent of US corn and cotton, 93 percent of soybeans, and 95 percent of sugar beets in the United States are genetically modified, Roundup Ready crops. Aside from weed protection, they say, another benefit of GM wheat would be to help combat crop loss due to a prolonged drought. While no incontrovertible research exists that proves GM crops are harmful, that argument quickly becomes irrelevant for wheat. America exports about 45 percent of its yield to Asia and Europe. The EU and twenty-six other countries including Japan at present ban or partially ban GMOs—genetically modified organisms. That potential loss of export business overshadows potential agricultural benefits, as was made clear in May 2013, when an Oregonian farmer discovered GM wheat in his field—the source remains uncertain—and notified the USDA. Oregon ships 90 percent of its soft wheat to Asia. Japan, Taiwan, and South Korea all refused to accept more shipments until assured that they were not genetically modified.

Josh Sosland, executive editor of *Milling & Baking News* in Kansas City, Missouri, says that without GM, "the future of wheat in America is in doubt." He speaks with authority: for ninety years his family has been the leading publisher of grain and milling industry information. "Even agnostics point out that people die from food poisoning every year but no one has ever become sick from GMOs. This boycott is nuts! they say. There's no science behind it."

To Borlaug in the past or to today's agri-scientists dealing with mass-hunger issues, debates about hypothetical alleged long-term consequences of GM or gluten sensitivity give way in an instant to larger, more urgent concerns. "You can't build a peaceful world on empty stomachs and human misery," Borlaug said in his final years, speaking for them all.

How can we take this in and make it relevant to our own lives? As average Americans we have options not available to people living in emerging nations. We have the luxury of deciding if a food choice may or may not agree with our metabolism or our personal values. To me Borlaug's single-minded quest for a solution to a world crisis puts my own dietary concerns into proper perspective—by comparison mine appear trivial and self-absorbed. It gives perspective as well to the debate about whether Borlaug's modern dwarf variety has created a massive increase in the ratio of gluten in wheat products. The argument serves Davis and his cohorts, even if prominent plant geneticists refute that theory.

At the same time, I recognize that the way dwarf hybrids have been manipulated by our country's grain industry since Borlaug's discovery renders it far less nutritious and far less interesting to eat than it need be. For most of us, the 93 percent without gluten issues, it represents no health threat, but so what? America's commercial wheat still lacks any sort of character. The agribusinesses in control of this commodity still put yield above all other considerations, even if they are not charged with feeding a starving nation. Flavor and nutritive value go by the wayside; no effort is made to cultivate heritage varieties or mill wheat to keep components intact. Enrichment adds back some but by no means all of the vitamins and minerals that get roller-milled out to cattle feeding troughs.

As an individual consumer, my way around the problem is to purchase flour from smaller boutique companies like King Arthur (see Appendix B) that care about the origin and treatment of the wheat they sell, and to buy baked goods from local artisans who labor to deliver all the gifts the grain has to offer. That may not be an option available to everyone, I fully understand, but if you do have the choice to experience the full enjoyment of whole fresh wheat, to take advantage of an opportunity that I, for one, do not take for granted, it will open up a new universe of taste and texture. And perhaps if enough of us make the case, we can actually influence the commercial bakeries to focus on real, nutritious whole grains instead of falling back on "enrichments" or chasing the latest dietary fad.

8

The Whole Truth

> How can a nation be called great if its bread tastes like Kleenex?
>
> —Julia Child

After six months of research I found that public opinion about wheat and my own expert-driven experience were moving farther apart day by day. Proponents of the gluten-free and Paleolithic diets continued to relegate anything and everything made from the grain to the status of toxic health risk and they seemed to be gaining ever more traction.

I knew exactly why: they hadn't yet found their way to Ponsford's Place in San Rafael, California, about twenty miles north of San Francisco. It's there that I find myself one warm, breezy late afternoon in August in the company of what I've come to call the Whole-Wheat West Coast Mafia. To my left sits one of the country's most popular writers on bread, Peter Reinhart; on the right, next to my wife, Bonnie, sits Janice Cooper, the executive director of the California Wheat Commission, and at a nearby table, Mark Shigenaga, a leading scientific researcher on gut flora, a.k.a. microbiota.

We are all gobbling up slices of nutty mocha-brown pizza baked to perfect toothy firmness as if this is the first meal we've been served after a yearlong fast. Toppings include fresh herbs, thin slivers of broccolini and yellow peppers draped with melted Fontina Val d'Aosta cheese, or razor thin slices of caramelized fennel and sweet onion interlaced with shaved Sicilian olives under a velvet ultrathin blanket of semisoft Trugole cheese.

Next to our small table a line has formed that extends out the door and down the block. We're in a working-class residential area, in a former freestanding barbershop converted into a compact two-room bakery owned and operated by a world-renowned baker, Craig Ponsford, and his wife, Diana Benner, a marine biologist.

Unassuming Ponsford's Place stands as ground zero for the burgeoning local Bay Area movement in whole-wheat artisan baking, and to Ponsford himself it represents a radical life and career change. In 1996 the baker's white-flour breads and pastries won a Gold Medal at the Coupe du Monde de la Boulangerie in Paris—the World Cup of Baking. The invitation-only competition, held every three to four years, draws teams from twelve countries across the globe and eighty thousand visitors. Mounted on one wall of Ponsford's Place is the apron he wore when he placed first at the event, signed by all of the other competing bakers. Little did he know, he says, what his future held in store—a total rejection of the white flour that brought him fame for his skills in laminating butter and dough and other ingredients into puffy croissants, brioche, and other delectable *Viennoiseries*. But when he fell out with his partners in a thriving boutique bakery he co-owned in Sonoma about a dozen years after his World Cup award, Ponsford stopped to consider what he enjoyed, and did not, about his craft. He loved the work itself, he realized, but not the medium.

"By then," he told me, "I'd had it with something I had no personal connection to. So one day in 2009—I distinctly remember the moment—I used white flour for the last time."

The magnitude of that decision for Ponsford—to produce no baked goods, neither croissants, turnovers, nor baguettes, nor ciabatta from any wheat that wasn't milled 100 percent whole—can hardly be overstated. At the top of his profession, performing baking feats that dazzled customers and international food writers and judges, his work no longer sparked his own interest or curiosity. There was also a philosophical basis to his decision. As Ponsford told an audience in 2013 at the International Association of Culinary Professionals in San Francisco, he realized, "A seed is a miracle. And when you take apart a wheat berry, it seems to kill it."

All fine and good, but a baker has to earn a living. Ponsford's Place? Not yet on the menu. "I knew nothing about whole grain," he told me. "I only knew I didn't want the sugar spike and crash of white flour ever again." Suddenly, for the first time in memory, Ponsford had nowhere to go and nothing to do. But he did have a friend who mattered—Joseph Vanderliet, an independent miller who got his start in the 1950s as a grain buyer for Archer Daniels. Vanderliet now operated his own whole-grain mill, Certified Foods, in Woodland, northwest of Sacramento.

"What's next for you?" Joe asked.

"I wish I knew," Ponsford answered.

To Vanderliet, that was not a satisfactory answer. He'd built Certified from scratch to mill organic wheat, corn, rice, and rye flour *his* way, and only his way, whole and intact. Watching Ponsford flounder about like a beached whale did not sit well with him. Vanderliet knew the baker to be as single-focused and uncompromising as he, his kind of perfectionist.

"Joe heard I was out on the street and offered me a little job to get my head out of my ass," Ponsford recalled. Little did he guess, he added, that Vanderliet's offer would lead him to reexamine everything he thought he knew about flour and baking. "I always just assumed you had to discard the undesirable parts of the kernel, the bitter germ and chunky bran, to get that airy texture. All my baking was 98 percent white flour."

Vanderliet offered Ponsford an opportunity to run Certified's test kitchen and soon after called him out when he heard Ponsford complaining about the difficulty of working with whole wheat, which absorbs more water and leavens entirely differently than white flour. "It's there for you to learn from," said Vanderliet, not a man who exhibits any patience for whining—as I was soon to discover on my own. Ponsford got the message, and within weeks he was busily adapting each of his white-flour formulas to suit the new tactile messages his whole-wheat dough transmitted during the mixing stage. Bakers think with their hands. Touch and feel determine elasticity, water absorption, leavening peculiarities—a host of specifics that vary through the seasons as humidity and temperature levels rise and fall. The best of them, like Ponsford, are dough whisperers.

We know, those of us gathered around the small table on this radiant August afternoon at his San Rafael bakery, downing Ponsford's exquisitely light but filling 100 percent whole-wheat pizzas. As a soothing marine breeze drifts in from nearby Richardson Bay, rays of fading summer sunlight slide over the western green and gold pillow hills and slant in through the two street-facing front windows. In one a fading sign reads, BE NICE OR LEAVE.

The bakery's odd location, along with the limited opportunity to sample its whole-wheat fare (Ponsford opens for business two days a week), only serves to escalate its cultlike status among the Bay Area's ardent foodies, who graze a gastronomical range that blankets about a hundred square miles from Berkeley in the east to Palo Alto in the south, north to Marin and beyond to Napa and Sonoma. Word spreads virally via social media. Judgments are made on the fly. One Chowhound member's mid-Ponsford-bite post reads: "Good lord . . . thanks. Don't have time to write more, but I'm having the savory turnover now and . . . it is one of the best things I've had this year—black-eyed peas, dandelion greens, arugula and four cheese!" A hymnal, an incantation shared by a choir of acolytes.

But perhaps the highest compliment comes from the man beside me, Peter Reinhart: after all, he wrote the book on pizza, the James Beard Award–winning *American Pie* by name. "This," he says, swallowing a last bite with a wolflish grin, "is heaven." Sometime back, Reinhart told his audience in a TED talk, "After forty years of knowing whole grains were a healthier option, we're tipping over and actually attempting to eat them. . . . We think of health foods as something we eat out of obligation, not out of passion."

These fragrant firm-but-chewy Ponsford creations tell a different story. They're part of my ongoing education. Sooner or later all abstract discussions about wheat and any other food source bow to sensory experiences; the food fails or succeeds not on the basis of lofty issues like nutritive value but primal impressions of taste, scent, and mouthfeel. What I'd learned was that good and good-for-you merge in whole-wheat items created with a full understanding of their performance properties, when fresh-milled to express their rich layered notes of fig, date, and, on occasion, spices like cardamom.

By now I'd met up with half a dozen more celebrity artisan bakers in the Bay Area, where a new Chad Robertson Farro Porridge–

Hazelnut Bread can generate the sort of fan frenzy devoted to a Brad and Angelina sighting in Hollywood. Like Craig Ponsford they all knew Joe Vanderliet's Certified Foods, and more specifically they praised his proprietary milling methods. I was eager to find out more and arranged a meeting.

The mill's small reception area looked out onto an expanse of shimmering sunflower and wheat fields. On one wall hung a large poster of the Joseph's Best whole-wheat flour bag, whose wide, vivid red border surrounds a large two-tone woodcut of a nineteenth-century granary, one that Jane Austen's Mr. Darcy might have galloped past on his horse as he paid a visit to the Bennet family. Perched on the sloping roof of the round lower building, which is shaped like a toadstool, sits a taller rectangular wooden structure, the grain hopper, fronted by a large windmill. The double-decker stone-ground mill evokes the feeling of a children's fable, yet it also appears to be, in its odd way, quaintly functional.

The intention clearly is to underscore the legacy of authenticity and integrity that distinguishes Certified Foods' whole-grain products, achieved utilizing the latest milling technology. Vanderliet in person conveyed the same sense of gravitas. The man I met when invited into his office stood at least six feet three inches, ramrod straight. Now in his early eighties, with a full head of hair, he maintained the focus and bearing of an alert, intense younger man.

"What do you know about wheat?" he asked me as I sat down. His steel-blue eyes met mine. "What do you know about flour? About farine?"

He leaned forward in his desk chair. "*Flour*, the word, came from *fleur*, or "flower" in French, so you've got two things going on, since it also can mean 'the finest,' as in '*fleur de farine*,' the finest part of the meal—the white endosperm, not the bran and germ, which were considered dirty, you following?" When Vanderliet fixes you with his piercing gaze and monitors for any signs of inattention, he spirits you back in time to that fiercely intelligent, autocratic college seminar professor who could constrict your bowels with one lift of a bushy eyebrow.

"As the process became mechanized, people lost their local millers. And I'll tell you something else these big giant roller operations did: they robbed those people of important minerals and vitamins they weren't getting any longer from the bran and germ."

"But what about enriching white flour by putting nutrients back in at the end?" I asked.

Joe V, as he's known to industry veterans, snorted and waved me off as if I were trying to sell him a dead donkey. "It's what they call 'reconstituted.' It's what I call bullshit! Once the seed's chemical bonds are broken, its antioxidants deteriorate. High heat from those rollers finishes them off."

The tagline of a print handout entitled "Certified Food's Guiding Philosophy" reads: "Whole wheat had a great fall and it can't be put back together again." That is, once the kernel is cracked like an egg, according to the copy, "no amount of fortification can return the balance of nutrients to the flour." A three-column chart on the last page compares the percentage of vitamins and minerals in whole-wheat flour versus refined and enriched flour. The latter two deliver only 5 percent of the vitamin E and less than half of just about everything else—zinc and manganese take the biggest hits. The only exceptions are the four enriched nutrients reintroduced by law, plus folate, added in 1998.

We were still less than five minutes into our meeting, and in the next five Joe filled me in on the history of Turkey Red, brought over in traveling trunks and kitchen crocks by those pacifist Russian Mennonite immigrants to the Plains States and Canada, where the croplands were similar to the Crimean Peninsula. He was about to expound on the two thousand or so miles of railroad track laid down to link grain elevators in Kansas when he must have picked up a sign of restlessness.

"There's more but you want to know about me and Certified."

"I do."

"I started as a grain buyer for Archer Daniels Midland Company back in the fifties, and by the 1980s I was running a terrific operation in Oakland for Montana Mills. It was the Mercedes-Benz of roller mills. One day a miller from Australia came by. I showed him around and he said to me, 'Have you ever thought about the nutritional value of what you're doing?' Just a question. I'd never thought about it. I was on top of the world at that time, but it stayed with me. I did some research and I was shaken."

For Vanderliet, that jolt of recognition proved profoundly disruptive. He had managed to survive World War II as a boy in the Netherlands, helping to feed his family by stealing chickens and garden vegetables at night; small at eight years old, he kept low to the ground so he wouldn't be picked up by the Nazi soldiers' searchlights. Taller boys, including his older brother, were captured and thrown into concentration camps. He'd also barely managed to avoid being conscripted into the Hitler Youth movement. After the war in the mid-'50s he made his way to Canada on a student visa. He was nineteen, with less than a hundred dollars in his pocket. One memory that stayed with him through all those years was the taste of a loaf of bread given to him by a farmer when he was scavenging food by night. "It was delicious, but more. It saved us from starving. My mother wept."

Years later, bread, which helped his family survive the trauma of wartime, provided his prestigious, well-paying position as plant manager in Oakland. But after that encounter with the visiting Australian, Vanderliet's research led him to take meetings with six of the highest executives in the industry. "The level of ignorance was astounding! They were pumping double bleach into their wheat to make it whiter than white. They had no idea of the effect nor any interest in learning." Although deeply troubled that the nutritious components of milled wheat (and corn) were not getting to the consumer, Joe still had to provide for his wife and five children, so he stayed in the corporate end of the wheat business until 1992, when he raised enough capital to start Certified Foods. His first mill came from West Kansas. The farmers who sold it to him also drove it out to California and installed it in two days with Vanderliet's modifications, and he was soon contracting with local wheat growers.

Over the years since then, he has perfected his own—and closely guarded—method of producing finely granulated wheat, rice, and rye flours. While stone milling grinds a kernel in a single pass that keeps bran, germ, and endosperm intact, it produces flour too coarsely ground to meet Vanderliet's demanding standards. He solved that problem by retooling components and adding a hammer-mill pass to his process, all the while maintaining a lower heat level in order to preserve the integrity of the nutrients. Touring the spotless facility with him, you see only massive pastel cylinders, while inside and well out of view, hammer rods and stones and, in last stage, rollers all work in synch to convert organic kernels into a fine flour that delivers Joe V's signature velvet whole wheat: for many experienced bakers, the texture is a revelation. Joseph's Best has none of the bitterness associated with the germ's fatty acids; in fact, it comes across as slightly sweet and brings to mind lightly roasted coffee and raw almonds. Vanderliet assures me that it degrades slowly, if at all, over six months or more when packaged.

While he remains tight-lipped about his proprietary methods—his reticence is legendary—industry veterans speculate that Certified achieves the combination of full whole-wheat nutrition, superior flavor, fine granulation, and long shelf life by coating the bran and germ with a thin layer of endosperm, or starch; that could explain how he neutralizes the rancidity of the oils while combining the antioxidants in the bran with the germ to stabilize its fats.

As I was about to leave a few hours later, Vanderliet handed me two five-pound bright red granary-illustrated flour bags. "You'll want to try this," he said, doing the steely-eyed thing again, but now with an unmistakable twinkle. "Probably more than once."

Stamping Out Advice

The Whole Grains Council, a nonprofit funded in part by Cargill, General Mills, and Kraft Foods, along with just about every one of our country's commercial bakers and millers, has a problem: the public's rejection of whole grains. Commodity millers provide less than 5 percent of their grain in whole-wheat form. Joe V is not stone-milling it and most consumers have no idea what wizards like Craig Ponsford can do with it, so it continues to be plagued by a serious image issue. I happened to catch a guest appearance by Michael Pollan on *The Colbert Report* to plug his 2013 book, *Cooked*. Challenged to come up with a quick healthful Friday night meal, Pollan recommended making whole wheat pasta. "Whole wheat pasta *sucks*!" cried Stephen

Colbert in a millisecond. That drew instantaneous loud laughter and sustained applause from the audience. Case sealed.

"The first time I ate organic whole-grain bread," Robin Williams once said, "I swear it tasted like roofing material." As a food product vying for supermarket shelf space, you do not want to be any famous comedian's punch line.

Local artisan bakers may be turning out delectable edibles, but in many areas of the country that still qualifies as a well-kept secret. While products made with 100 percent whole grain often deliver both taste and nutrition, and consumer patterns are slowing shifting in their direction, they carry a lot old baggage.

For decades, we associated 100 percent whole wheat with those anchor-weight dense hippie loaves of the sixties and seventies. In the absence of activated gluten they seemed to compress and shrink rather than expand. "Door stops" was a familiar description. Today, whole wheat invariably makes the list of intelligent food choices that win over our rational minds but not our pleasure-seeking palates. In this ongoing skirmish tongue receptors can be counted on to trump brain receptors.

Cynthia Harriman knows all about that. As the Whole Grains Council's director of Food and Nutrition Strategies, it is her job to oversee the Whole Grain Stamp program and fill the Whole Grains website with helpful, interesting information.

If you accept the premise that you'll find very little that is negative about wheat on the site, it offers an excellent menu of recipes and much more, along with an exhaustive listing of the grams of whole wheat in every bread, cake mix, and flour product made in America, it seems.

Harriman is especially proud of the stamp. It comes in two

flavors—the 100 Percent Stamp, for products where all the grain is whole grain, and the Basic Stamp, for products made with a mix of whole and refined grain—and it appears on more than ten thousand products in forty-four countries. Both are intended to help consumers increase whole-grain consumption.

I know, as you do, that we're all encouraged to eat three servings or about 3 to 4 ounces of whole grains a day as a way of preventing or combating strokes, coronary disease, diabetes, high blood pressure, obesity, and certain types of cancer in addition to lowering cholesterol and avoiding constipation. The medical community generally acknowledges these health benefits, excepting the non-gluten lobby that lumps whole and refined wheat together as a deadly duo.

The FDA doesn't do much to clarify a confusing conundrum for consumers by requiring that 51 percent of the total weight of the product be whole grain to display a whole-grain stamp. But at least 40 percent of that weight is water. The industry itself could let us know exactly what percent of the balance of dried solid grains are whole.

According to Livestrong and dozens of other sources, 100 percent whole wheat does not precipitate a sudden glucose boost when absorbed by the bloodstream. On the glycemic index (GI), the scale from zero to 100 that ranks the speed with which the carbohydrates in any given food causes a rise in blood sugar, with pure glucose set at 100, it comes in at 51. A study by the Harvard School of Public Health points out that a lower GI, under 55, reduces the risk of type 2 diabetes and assists with weight loss. But Harriman disputes that. She argues that more reliable studies put all commercial whole-wheat breads—100 percent included—at about 71 on the GI.

Public health professor David R. Jacobs and his team at the University of Minnesota reviewed seventeen studies that consistently found a 20 to 40 percent reduction in the long-term risk of atherosclerotic cardiovascular diseases and type 2 diabetes in 100 percent whole-grain consumers compared to those who rarely eat those foods. As much as 75 percent of the phytochemicals in plants that produce beneficial health results are lost in the refining process.

A pivotal difference is nutrient density, more nutrients and phytochemicals for fewer calories. A nutrient-dense normal serving of 100 percent whole-wheat pasta or whole-grain bread will deliver, for instance, two to five times as much vitamin E; you'd need to eat an additional 320 calories derived from white flour to acquire the same amount of that vitamin, the equivalent of a thirty-three-pound weight gain every year. Whole grains rank halfway in micronutrients between raw leafy vegetables at the high end of nutritional density and refined grains such as processed cereals and sugar sweets on the bottom rungs.

These benefits on paper should sway us all. But still only one person in twenty between nineteen and fifty years old actually comes anywhere close to consuming the recommended daily quantity of whole grains. On average, Americans eat less than one third of the suggested daily total.

Every serving is listed in grams on the Basic Stamp, to be consistent with what the FDA requires on the Nutrition Facts Panel. The stamp tells us to eat 48 grams or more of whole grains daily; apparently we're supposed to know a gram equals 1/28 of an ounce. "We'd much rather talk servings," says Harriman, "but for complex reasons the FDA and USDA make that impossible." (To complicate matters for the council, in January 2013 a Harvard School of Public Health study reported that these boldly stamped baked goods can be loaded with sneaky sugar and calories, even while acknowledging that they deliver 46 percent more fiber. In Harriman's view, Harvard sensationalized the results, but both she and the stamp survived.)

The major health benefit of 100 percent whole grains with bran intact we all know: fiber. It's been pitched for more than a century as a way to avoid constipation, of course, but there's more to it, I learned. It's also the meal of choice for our most friendly intestinal bacteria, not a guess I would have made.

Strategic Weapon

A hot topic for scientific study these days is the proper care and feeding of our microbiome, or gut flora. Fiber intake is critical to keeping that bacteria well fed, scientists recently discovered, and well-fed bacteria help in lowering body weight and alleviating obesity-induced chronic inflammation. They also perform related anti-inflammatory functions. Researchers now know that fiber plays a potential therapeutic role in treating allergic diseases and lowering vulnerability to asthma attacks. Too little fiber can starve friendly bacteria, not a good thing because those same bacteria begin to eat us—that is, the mucus lining of our large intestine. In addition, a high-fiber diet reduces the risk of internal blood clots, thrombosis, and cholesterol-related conditions. We've lost diversity in our microbiota, which is crucial to maintaining health, says Justin Sonnenburg, a microbiologist at the Stanford School of Medicine and coauthor of *The Good Gut*. He speculates that our Western diet provides us with five to ten times less daily fiber than our ancestors consumed. Dietary fibers, like those in sourdough whole wheat bread, help to add that diversity.

Dr. Robert Lustig in *Fat Chance* calls fiber "the most misunderstood weapon in our nutritional arsenal." The outer layers of wheat bran form a barrier of dead insoluble cells, fibrous material that defends against seed degradation. Our systems put that plant strategy to good use. Insoluble fiber is roughage, and roughage hangs around in the alimentary canal long enough to give us a feeling of fullness when we eat, so that we don't stuff ourselves as we might otherwise. The water it absorbs—and it absorbs up to three times its weight—adds bulk to our stool. That creates pressure on the walls of our colon, signaling the need for daily elimination.

It's still promoted to the over-seventy crowd as a sure cure for regular bowel movements, Lustig reminds us, while its more important value lies in preventing colon cancer and diverticulitis. Fiber's importance, he adds, should also embrace its role as half the antidote to the obesity pandemic. In conversation, as in print, Lustig presents his arguments with absolute authority, ready in a heartbeat to drop his guillotine on any conclusion not backed by "real science"—it must be both replicable and verifiable. "At UCSF [the teaching hospital where he practices in San Francisco] we have a saying: 'In God we trust, everyone else has to show the data.'"

His data tells him that fiber's impact depends on whether it is soluble (in water) or insoluble. If soluble it slows digestion and ferments to gas in the colon; if insoluble, as in whole wheat, it has a laxative effect and speeds the passage of waste through your gut.

Both function together as a hair catcher in your shower drain, in the vivid metaphor Lustig uses. Insoluble fiber forms the latticework; soluble fiber bridges the gaps—and in effect it adds finer netting. In tandem, the two slow the rate of food metabolized by the liver, allowing the liver time to properly function. Refined grains stripped of bran and germ, as opposed to whole, lack fiber and micronutrients. As a result, processed grains cause an overflow of serum glucose in the liver. But "whole" does not always mean whole, Lustig recognizes, not when FDA and the Institute of Medicine (IOM) strip away the real meaning of the word and leave behind the starchy endosperm of a nutrient-poor definition. More specifically, reducing "whole" to mean a minimum of 51 percent in the IOM definition, Lustig remarks diplomatically, "leaves much to be desired." There's nothing diplomatic in his tone.

I admit to an instinctive distrust of any institute or regulatory agency that encourages double-talk, but the good news for me at the moment was that I could leave all of that behind. It was time to pay a visit to another part of the forest, where the artisan wheatheads gambol around wood-fire bread ovens under a starry firmament and plant seeds that become strands of funny-looking grain nobody's grown for a century. It was time to move back into the future of American wheat.

9
Flour Power

> The smell of good bread baking, like the sound of lightly flowing water, is indescribable in its evocation of innocence and delight.
>
> —M. F. K. Fisher

You recall Joe Vanderliet, the miller whose cocked eyebrow brooked no flirtation with inattention or ignorance. I met up again with Joe V a few months after our initial meeting, at an event that I've come to call Wheatstock, as in Woodstock. Officially it billed itself as a gathering of Bay Area and Northern California artisan local grain mavens from grower to chef to celebrity baker to prominent microbial scientist. The sound of steam hissing from bread ovens provided the flour-power music that brought us all to this updated version of Max Yasgur's farm on a Sunday morning in March 2014. The panelists and about 120 attendees from food writer to trend spotter to home baker convened upstairs at Oliveto, a venerable Oakland Italian restaurant owned by Maggie and Bob Klein, the host, who started Community Grains in 2007 more or less out of desperation. Klein could not locate fresh, intensely flavorful organic durum or whole-wheat flour for the Oliveto dishes he and his executive chef wanted to create. Klein's standards of excellence were absurdly high, but so, too, were his energy, passion, and determination. Out of his lengthy, often exasperating search for what I've come to call true wheat, his new company, Community Grains, was born.

The striving for deep flavor and resilient texture that spawned the local Bay Area grain movement now ripples across the country, primarily on both coasts from Skagit Valley in upstate Washington to South Brooklyn to North Carolina. But on this Sunday morning Oliveto is at its California epicenter, and Bob Klein embodies both its ambitious spirit and its grounded pragmatism, with a large helping of maniacal advocate tossed in to spice the blend. He took on whole grain as a secular religion: never rent asunder bran, germ, and endosperm, you can just about hear Klein preaching at a pulpit as an unlikely spiritual descendant of Sylvester Graham, for thou shalt pay a fearsome price in body, soul, and spirit.

But in reality Bob Klein never preaches, he enthuses. Like the best salesmen everywhere, he rarely raises his voice. One on one, with low-throttle conviction, he lays out the argument for how and why legions of people who care about the welfare of the planet we live on, and their own health, will make their way back in time to local whole wheat and corn, organically grown and milled within a hundred miles or so from where they live and eat—by agricultural standards, close by, within the same region or state, not half a continent or an ocean away.

Setting aside eating enjoyment for the moment, energy and natural resource consumption add muscle to Klein's assertion. Pound for pound, Elizabeth Kolbert points out in "Stone Soup," her *New Yorker* overview of the current Paleo diet trend, beef production uses ten times as much or more water than wheat and, calorie for calorie, close to twenty times as much energy. Your next flank steak also contributes to global warming; livestock are a major source of greenhouse-gas emissions. By one analysis in the *American Journal of Clinical Nutrition* referenced by Kolbert, a pound of beef produces polluting gas emissions that are the equivalent of driving forty-five miles, while a pound of wheat totals only one mile.

A local grain economy does not transform waste into preservation on its own, as Klein readily admits, but it redefines an industry that leaves us as daily consumers—about 4.5 billion people eat wheat every day around the globe—in a state of ignorance about the origin and processing of the food we're getting more than 20 percent of our calories from. One of local grain's many virtues, he argues, is transparency. "Each of our products," Klein says, "carries a specific history we're proud to share." In that spirit, every box of Community Grains dried whole-wheat pasta arrives with a description of the kind of wheat used, where it was grown, also when harvested and milled. Bonnie (no longer gluten-free by then; I'll get to that, trust me) and I tried a hard amber durum fusilli ("spindles" in Italian) grown in West Sonoma by Front Porch Farms, we learned, and stone-milled at a low temperature at Certified Foods by Joe Vanderliet, who has teamed up with Klein to produce specialty pasta and flour for Community Grains.

Compared to $1.95 De Cecco or Barilla, the box we bought at Whole Foods was expensive, about $5, a sensible reason for skipping past it as you move down the aisle, but when we boiled and ate that fusilli, price became an afterthought. Its earthy, lightly herbal complexity and chewy yet smooth texture combined to produce an exquisite, rare eating experience. Community Grains' website now features "Identity Preserved" pastas that name the wheat variety—Durum Iraq, for instance—and clarify relevant terms like *landrace*. That term singles out locally adapted, naturally evolving varieties of plants like heritage grains (as true for the Iraq) as opposed to varieties developed by seed companies. TMI? Maybe to you and me, but not too much information for Klein. After the conference I would trace that Durum Iraq back to its origins, an organic farm called Full Belly in the farmlands near Sacramento. There is a vast learning gap to bridge, as he frequently points out. Basically we know nothing about the pasta we eat except for the name of its shape, country of origin, and generic variety, semolina or whole wheat.

Someday Klein hopes to offer that same purity-plus-pleasure equation, along with the nutritional benefits of whole grains to consumers at a more affordable retail price. Organic tomatoes provide his most favored analogy. In the seventies, he explains, we ate tasteless, watery, store-bought red rubber balls that were a vegetable equivalent of refined white flour—shorn of all identifying or nutrifying traits. As local boutique growers introduced us to organic heritage tomato varieties, Black Cherokee and others, at their farmer's market stalls and to subscribers to CSAs (boxes containing community-supported agricultural produce and fruits), we gradually became converts. Newly acquainted with intensely delicious flavors, we soon formed an eager consumer base. We're now willing to spend up to $5 or $6 a pound to enjoy our favorite heirlooms, and some of us fetch them at Walmart and Trader Joe's at lower cost. Proving its worth, a niche product crossed over to mainstream.

That clean trajectory may elude local wheat, since the grain requires threshing, storing, and milling, more costly and labor-intensive steps to get to market, but there are enough potential parallels to light up the pathway to future success for an entrepreneurial visionary like Klein. While he's been described as a pied piper of the whole-grain movement, he comes across more accurately as the piper's avuncular mentor. Now in his mid-sixties with an expansive gourmand waistline, full gray bristly beard, glasses, ruminative demeanor, and slight slouch, he could pass in his sweater vest as the fusty dean of an Ivy League philosophy department. But he wouldn't last a day. He'd be tossed off campus for torching all the breadbaskets in the college cafeteria if he found them filled with white-flour breads and rolls; he'd call for a boycott until a decent supply of whole-wheat focaccia, miches, ciabatta, and pane pugliese arrived.

Klein knows that building an infrastructure to get Community Grains' products and others like it to interested consumers requires a distribution network not yet in place, even if Whole Foods has successfully tested Klein's Community Grains pasta and is increasing its shelf space in some metropolitan regions.

Klein's most useful gift, as I've come to observe, is his ability to attract, inspire, and involve talented, energized, well-connected people to his cause. To succeed he needs them all: a pool that includes small heritage wheat growers, millers, celebrated chefs and bakers, nationally acclaimed journalists, scientists publishing in peer-reviewed journals; then, too, he has to team with large grocery chain baked-good buyers, knowing that farmer's markets on their own are only a first step. No better example comes to mind than the ten panelists he's lined up for this Sunday conference, which sold out in less than a day. In addition to Pollan, who also teaches in UC Berkeley's Journalism Department between books and is a close Klein ally, the morning lineup includes nutritional scientists Mark Shigenaga and David Killilea from CHORI and whole-wheat nutritional epidemiologist David Jacobs, who analyzes health and disease patterns in defined populations.

I know what you're thinking. We gave up our Sunday morning

paper and toasted bagel for epidemiology? Nobody in the audience, however, seems to be fidgeting. We get that for the first time in memory American wheat is speaking with a voice all its own, and we want to know what it has to say. After tasting samples of numerous baskets of deliciously rich, crunchy-chewy, fresh whole-wheat wedges made from local sources by the artisan bakers in attendance, we're eager to absorb details and sure to trade opinions and experiences during the lunch break. Video documentary producer and writer Maggie Beidelman will later capture the tenor of the event in the headline of her coverage: "What if Everything You Knew About Grains Was Wrong?"

Microbiologist Mark Shigenaga starts things off by contrasting white flour, which he argues can produce hangover symptoms and a "food coma," to eating whole grains. "We see it in test tubes, the enzymes in our saliva break down white and whole-wheat flour completely differently, it's day and night. White all at once, whole in measured amounts, so that it has little impact on our gut walls and immunological systems." Those beneficial bacteria in our gut walls, he added, also love the fiber in whole wheat. And why is it so many Americans who have a hard time with domestic wheat products tolerate bread with no problems in Europe? "It's in the difference in wheat quality and structure. They're eating wheats milled in a way that's similar to Joe Vanderliet's methods, often, which is why they don't stress out our digestive systems."

Pollan, in a big-picture mode, tells us that Klein and a coterie of local grainers around the country "are asking us to join a new civilization." That gets my attention. This could be a country club I'd like to join, even if it would have me as a member. The bread would be delicious. Local breeding and milling, Pollan continues, creates an entirely different microbial culture that can't be duplicated in wheats grown by the current industrial wheat complex. Those strains, with harder, bitterer bran and swollen endosperms, are bred to serve the engineering design specifications of the mill's rollers as a delivery system for pure white flour. One set shears off that hard bran in large chunks.

As I scan the room and take in the palpable enthusiasm of audience members including luminaries like Harold McGee, the author of *On Food and Cooking*, an immensely informative classic on the science and lore of all things edible, I'm struck yet again by the schizophrenic nature of wheat in America today. It is killing us, some like William Davis and David Perlmutter avow. Or nurturing, rewarding, and fortifying us, according to folks at this gathering. I doubt that there is another non-narcotic plant anywhere that elicits such extreme contradictory conviction.

After many months on the prowl it has become clear to me that putting aside all else just for the moment, those anti-wheat crusaders may be missing the best part of the story. By focusing exclusively on the Borlaug inheritance, a carbo-saturated flour derived from a nitrogen-boosted, generic field crop, wheat's detractors have cheated themselves of the pleasure of exploring flavors and nutritional benefits readily available from the same grain when bred, farmed, and processed to accentuate its strengths. There are heritage varieties out there that taste like chocolate, that give off the scent of earthy woodlands after a spring rain—who knew?

No one I've met understands or executes on these strengths and surprises with more assurance than afternoon panelist Stephen Jones, director of Washington State University's Research and Extension Center at Mount Vernon in Skagit Valley, north of Seattle.

Jones breeds wheats at the WSU eighty-acre experimental farm that I'd visited a few months prior to Klein's conference; his plants grow in a staggering array of different lines—forty thousand wheat varieties in all. A large rangy man with the strong chin and rugged features of a frontier homesteader in a classic Western, Jones employs advanced technology like molecular cytogenetics to further the art and science of Old World breeding. One of his hybrids, by way of example, is Barber wheat, named for Dan Barber. co-owner and executive chef of Blue Hill at Stone Barns in Westchester, New York. Jones works with masterful chefs like Barber to learn what they look for in flavor, performance, and texture, and translates that into genetic coding.

For Barber, Jones's expertise opened up unexplored territory. Barber had never before thought of wheat as alive, fresh, and certainly not as a grain that could be custom-bred. "Wheat arrived at our restaurant kitchen as dead powder," he told a symposium of chefs in 2013. But when a *Time* magazine journalist introduced Barber to the seeds of a flavorful heritage wheat grown only in one village in Northeastern Spain, Aragon 03, by name, and Barber showed the seeds to Jones, the breeder's immediate response was, "Let me cross this and breed it for you on our farm."

Today, Barber wheat—with an apricot flavor and a delightful wet-hay aroma, he says—is one of those forty thousand experimental varieties. It helps that Jones makes bread at home and appreciates the qualities bakers look for. He's the rare gastronome who also knows his way around a genome. At Klein's gathering of the clan Jones took on a familiar topic. As a geneticist, he told the audience, he knew that despite growing "tasteless, soulless" modern wheat and refusing to rotate crops, thereby killing the soil, industrial agribusiness farmers were not producing kernels with higher amounts of gluten. "There's been a change," he continued, "but it's in the extra gluten, like vital gluten, a concentrate now commonly added into multigrain commercial doughs to keep them crumbling apart."

Panelist Chad Robertson, whose Tartine Bakery in San Francisco draws crowds that stand in line an hour or longer for the scant two hundred–plus loaves he bakes daily, talked about a recent Scandinavian trip that introduced him to a variety of older Nordic grains whose flavors "totally blew my mind." Young, handsome, and now a celebrity author of three bread books, Robertson maintains a guileless "way cool, dude!" attitude he transposed into baking from his other passion, surfing. The way Tartine decided to introduce whole wheat to its customers, he said, was through its cookies, and it worked: "Everyone loves them."

Panelist Matt Mestemacher, bakery coordinator for Whole Foods in Northern California, picked up on that. "We tested local California grown wheat in ice cream sandwiches first," he said, "and we didn't tell anyone. When we surveyed our customers, they loved the nuttiness. Then we told them it was stone-ground whole wheat. There was a typical look of total disbelief."

That led Whole Foods to produce its own whole-wheat chocolate chip cookies. "We sold fifty-five thousand in three weeks," he told the audience.

Klein, a few seats away at the panelist's table, jerked his head in Mestemacher's direction. "Did you say '*fifty-five thousand*'?"

It quickly became clear, said the Whole Foods buyer, that true wheat has a large potential following but that it won't make any sort of profound statement until there's a robust and reliable infrastructure in place. By my reckoning, Whole Foods may take a pioneering position across the country in initiating connections with local growers, millers, and bakers, but these products need to be readily accessible elsewhere, too, perhaps not through supermarket chains but at outlets that extend in a variety of directions beyond farmer's markets. Food scientists will ultimately determine if 100 percent whole-wheat items present less of a hazard to gluten-sensitives than do commoditized white-flour versions. They have already analyzed its slower rate of absorption, and lower glucose level, in the bloodstream.

To me, listening in as an average interested consumer, successful mainstream marketing remains the challenge that will either be met or, if not, consign the local grain economy to an asterisk in the locavore movement. I was probably taking home the wrong message, but I found it dispiriting that both Robertson and Mestemacher promoted cookies as ideal fare for entry-level whole-wheat acceptance, something in the order of a baby pool as an inducement to plunging into the deep water. I'm a great fan of cookies, but I'd like to believe that nutritional whole wheat does not need to be propped up or shilled in order to find a ready audience. On the other hand, I did hear Stephen Colbert's universal squeal of protest, loud and clear. He's never chowed down on locally grown whole-wheat pasta, for sure. Nor the luscious dark chewy grains we sampled and ate as morning muffins and sandwich bread at the Community Grains Conference. That, however, is not the 100 percent whole wheat America knows and shuns—not yet, at any rate.

If things are to change significantly, I reasoned, that will probably mean winning the hearts and minds (and tummies) of children, and quite possibly starting with cookies. Klein at one point mentioned his recent visit to a nearby school where students were testing whole-grain products. The notion stayed with me. I contacted Janice Cooper, executive director of the California Wheat Commission, for help, which she generously provided by leading me to Fat Cat Scones. The company's owners, she explained, might be amenable to letting me tag along on a taste test they conduct for some of their products in a public school classroom.

By then I'd listened to well-intentioned adults touting the virtues of local whole wheats that as yet remain unobtainable to most of us. But what about the wheat that most American kids are likely to eat at home or at school? Recent changes in federal health improvement regulations now require school districts to shift away from processed to real foods in student snacks and lunches. The concept, of course, is to introduce children to nutritious whole wheat and other whole foods at a young age, while malleable, encouraging them to adopt healthful choices as a lifelong habit. Is that simply wishful thinking? I'm guessing that it probably is, based on my own boyhood devotion to junk food. Still, I've heard rumors that times are in fact changin' mostly because the things that are good for us are being made in ways that are actually appealing to young appetites. I'll believe it when I see it, so I set off to find out for myself.

Show, Eat, and Tell

A few weeks after the conference I'm standing in a sixth-grade classroom in a blue-collar neighborhood of Sacramento beside Erik Finnerty, co-owner of Fat Cat Scones and room teacher Karin Springer. Finnerty has come to the Del Paso Manor Elementary School on a Friday afternoon with boxes of Fat Cat energy bars and cookies in tow, several flavor options of each. They meet the stringent USDA guidelines for fruit and grain servings, along with a recent federal law requiring that at least 51 percent of the flour be whole wheat. Finnerty could be walking into bedlam—these eleven-year-olds are about an hour away from spring recess. As any teacher knows, on the last day before vacation your students are racehorses in the starting gate.

You can feel the throbbing of hoofbeats in the stalls and at the sound of the dismissal bell they're primed to bolt through the open windows and sprint across the schoolyard to freedom, or so it seems. But Springer, clearly a pro, keeps calm control over her class; the boys and girls in this multiracial public school room listen attentively to Finnerty's instructions. For most of the next hour, this class will be his focus group. The rating sheets Finnerty passes ask the students to check one of three boxes for each product: Love, Maybe, and No Love. He hopes to accomplish two goals: to find out which of these whole-wheat products the class prefers; and to gauge how whole wheat measures up to white flour as a first preference.

"I want you to mark each one with what you think of it and then write why, in the space below. There are no free rides—you've got to tell me why you like it or don't. Think about texture and taste. I specifically want to know what you think about the whole wheat. The first is our Banana Chocolate Chip Farmers Market Bar. We buy the bananas, we let them sit around until they turn brown, that's when they're most flavorful, and then we puree them. There's nothing canned in any of these."

I admire Erik's approach. He doesn't talk down to the class; he's all business.

"Who eats whole-wheat bread at home?" he asks while the bars are being handed out. Just about everyone's hand raises.

"Who eats white bread?" I ask. A few scattered hands. I'm surprised; I expected white to dominate, or at least a more even distribution.

While the sixth graders smell, then bite into his banana bars, Erik gives them a quick overview of the "junkiness" of processed foods—the kind he describes as ones that make you fatter, not healthier. I scan the room to see who's paying attention, and I'm reminded that as an adult, you rarely know for sure until a smart question comes out of nowhere from a kid who seemed to be dozing off. Erik hands out three more samples, two cookies and two bars in all, none made with any preservatives. Taking their food-testing assignment seriously, many of the students sniff, make a note, then bite and make another note. When he surveys the class for flavors they've picked up, he gets back a long list of spices including nutmeg.

Polling the students on the two breakfast bars, Finnerty learns that they overwhelmingly prefer the banana bar to the second choice, flavored with pumpkin and cinnamon. "Too dry," the class agrees. No deliberations needed: they know in a flash what they like, and don't.

I take advantage of a short break after all four products have been tested to ask if anyone knows why whole wheat is better for you.

"White bread has more sugar," one girl answers.

"Whole wheat's got more fiber," a boy answers. He's not sure why that's good for you.

"It's minimally processed," another boy offers. "No bleaches."

Erik jumps in to add that it has more protein—a building block of life, he explains.

"Who can taste the whole wheat in these?" I ask. Five or six hands shoot up. "Who likes the taste of white-wheat cookies better?" Two hands shoot up out of about thirty students.

"Would you know that these are healthier than regular cookies and bars?" Erik asks, collecting their ballots. About 80 percent of the class couldn't tell one from the other. He explains to the class that he travels all around the country to food service shows where "75 percent of the products there are crud. They're made by big companies that are worried about how they can feed kids for cheap, they're not worried about quality."

Then, he adds, there are companies like Fat Cat. "We use real ingredients," he adds, "and they cost a little more. But you get what you pay for in this world."

As we were winding down one girl asks me, "What is your go-to inspirational quote?"

I stop to ponder that for a moment: "Never think you can't do anything, because you can always do it if you really want to." I have no idea where that came from.

"Who said it?" she demands.

"I did. I just made it up."

"No way!"

Apparently I've broken a rule: the quote has to come from someone famous, like Yoda.

A few minutes later, right before the bell, I ask Callie, seated in the front row and someone who's been actively participating in the discussion, why she says she won't eat processed foods. She thinks for a moment.

"They're like plastic surgery," she answers. "They hide all the wrinkles until you can't tell what's real and what's not."

Super-Tasters

If future generations of Americans embrace whole wheat with anything like genuine enthusiasm, that will most likely come about as a melding of early exposure in and out of school with a broadening retail distribution of tastier, more enticing, and more nutritious versions produced by local artisan bakers.

Suppliers like Finnerty and Tony Van Rees, Finnerty's partner and Fat Cat's executive chef, seem primed to play an important role. I met with them at their Fat Cat plant on the same day I visited Del Paso Elementary. By then I'd done a personal sampling of the four items the students rated. They were sweet but not cloying, filled with soft fruit chunks, thicker and less dense than energy bars, with a soft, cake-like texture. I didn't pick up pronounced flavor differences among them. Above all, they left a fresh taste behind, with no lingering off notes.

"Kids are super-tasters," Erik told me. "They have way more tongue receptors than we do, which is why we dump hot sauce on eggs and they don't. So you have to deliver food they want to eat. And hope you get support from their parents at home, otherwise Doritos win and whole grains lose. People may be scared of whole wheat, but then they have a visceral bread moment at an artisan bakery. They taste the crunchy crust and tell you, Wow, this is so amazing—and that filters down to their children."

"And how do the school districts you sell to make their decisions?"

"It's a moving target, because Congress is always changing the USDA requirements, and we have to be compliant to compete. But sooner or later it comes down to money. The school district's goal is to increase average daily participation to get a higher rate of reimbursement from the feds. And there's now a supper program as well in lower-income areas. So for us to do well, we have to be one of the reasons they get their participation up for every meal."

Fat Cat, Finnerty continues, buys all of its California whole-wheat flour from Joe Vanderliet's Certified Foods, about twenty miles away. "It's mild, it's mellow, with a good mouthfeel and texture; the kids like it—we tested fifteen or more flours before we made our choice. Most of our products are 60 to 100 percent whole grain."

Selling to local hotel restaurants, Finnerty and Van Rees started out as wholesale baking partners while still students at UC Santa Barbara. Now in their late thirties, they haven't entirely abandoned the spirit of those laid-back college days. Finnerty's vanity license plate reads SCONER, a clever play on stoner that also happens to identify his vocation. Until recently his ride was a bright orange boxy Honda Element that looked more at home on the beach than the boulevard. Trained as a pastry chef, Van Rees after graduation came up with a formula for frozen scones made in the softer European style; working out of Erik's garage, they launched Fat Cat. Their edge in competing with Pillsbury and other "big boys," says Van Rees, is that their school cookies and bars don't taste like cardboard. "Meanwhile," says Finnerty, "Cargill and the others use hard white whole wheat—it's processed to smithereens."

What he's referring to is an increasingly popular, newer cross-bred class of hard bread wheat with tannish white—not red—bran, whose flavor is milder since it does not contain the strongly flavored tannins found in red wheat. Hard white makes up the majority of wheat grown in Australia. It came to the United States in the 1970s and now accounts for 10 to 15 percent of our total crop. It's a popular choice for pizza dough. The original incentive, says the Whole Wheat Council, was to reverse a sharp decline in US wheat exports. For school sales, it meets government whole-wheat regulations while offering the bland flavor and color associated with all-purpose white flour.

Perception is reality, Finnerty says, for kids. "If they look at a lemon cookie that's traditionally white, and instead it's brown whole wheat, they freak." But both he and Van Rees trust that, even so, Fat Cat's full-flavor "real and pure" approach is right in line with changing USDA regulations. They've now expanded to seventeen states. The revelation for Van Rees, when they tested Joseph's Best from Certified Foods, was that the wheat had a distinctive flavor. "It has a delicious quality to it but one that I was not totally familiar with. I never really tasted wheat although I'd been making bread professionally all these years."

Like most of us, I thought to myself. As eleven-year-old Callie put it, that's what happens when wheat producers hide all its wrinkles until you can't tell what's real and what's not.

10

Mastering the $158 Loaf

> To be sensual, I think, is to respect and rejoice in the force of life . . . and to be present in all that one does, from the effort of loving to the breaking of bread.
>
> —James Baldwin, *The Fire Next Time*

There was one thing missing from all the research I had done to date: me—not as a reporter with a license to chill, but as a hands-on, roll-up-the-sleeves, work-up-a-sweat dough slinger. Oh yeah, tussling with wet flour on its way to becoming a loaf of bread is hard work, or so I'd heard and seen. Mixing by hand, that is, not sitting around watching it rise in the oven or flicking on a bread machine. Somewhere between viewing golden rows of wheat stalks dancing in the wind and breathing in the toasty aromas of baking ovens as I visited growers and bakers, I became enthralled with the notion of producing my own homemade organic bread by hand from scratch, including the starter, the doughy wild-yeast-and-lactic-bacteria concoction that ignites the fermentation engine. (Getting that starter to bubble up with escaping carbon dioxide gas and emit its signature vinegary scent I'll take up in Chapter 15.) Since the story of wheat is the story of bread and pasta, I owed it to my reader and myself, I reasoned, to develop an intimate relationship with my subjects.

Bonnie, when I told her my plan, had her own concerns. As wife and astute companion, she had been with me through decades of winemaking. She'd seen me mucking out fermentation tanks at four in the morning during crush, covered from head to foot in wrinkled grape skins; she'd watched me hover on a plank many feet up in the air over an open tank punching down thick caps of solid grape matter with a tool that looked like a metal toilet plunger on steroids. Also, she remembered an episode in which, armed with a thief, or glass siphon, I climbed up and down an extended ladder in a barrel room, glass in hand, to taste from more than thirty barrels stacked six high on metal racks for an upcoming blending session. The concrete ground twenty feet down from the highest perch was dotted with dark red splotches where I'd spit out my samples all afternoon after gurgling. There was nothing unusual about the session except that I got so involved that I lost track of time and was startled when suddenly the barrel room went pitch-black and a metal door slammed shut. The cellar master, not knowing I was high up in the rafters, locked me in and went home for the evening. That began a long, arduous trail of mishaps that got me back to our house four hours late for a dinner party.

"You can sometimes get a little carried away," she remarked gingerly.

No worries, I assured her, this comes down to following simple recipes, called formulas because they're so exact. And the wheat does all the work. You mix and it ferments while you sleep. Presto!

Three months into her gluten-free, neck-tension-loosening food regimen, my wife was losing interest fast. Wheat, sweet or sour, wasn't on her menu.

By then I knew whose bread-making instructions I planned to follow. On a baker's recommendation I'd picked up a copy of Andrew Whitley's *Bread Matters*. Scanning the first few pages, I found myself engrossed in the Englishman's eccentric yet authoritative blend of history, recipes, knowing tips, and barely suppressed fury at the nutritional price extracted by Britain's industrial bread-baking companies for their empty-calorie, additive-loaded products. Well-known in the UK for his relentless determination to improve its breads and help to a build local grain economy, Whitley created one of its first organic artisan bakeries in the seventies and cofounded the Real Bread Campaign whose large stamp on a loaf bag assures the consumer that the baker uses no artificial additives or processing aids. In *Bread Matters* Whitley offers an impassioned, detailed critique of England's version of Wonder Bread, developed in 1961 through the Chorleywood Bread Process; this is still the method of choice, he reports, for 80 percent of the UK's sliced breads. Wheat growers pump up their crops with massive doses of nitrogen to boost head size for more endosperm. Chorleywood's nutritional and flavor deficiencies led him to create England's first brick-oven-baked whole-grain breads.

Whitley devotes six crammed pages to the Chorleywood ingredients, a virtual chemistry lab in a loaf. Emulsifiers include mono- and diacetyl tartarics for loaf volume and crumb softness and the inevitable compounds intended to send the dough sliding unimpeded on its merry way in record time. Chorleywood's supporters—and there are many—point to its low cost and long shelf life. Whitley is not among them. Under a column titled "What's the Problem?" he spells out the issues associated with each ingredient—the most common being "no nutritional benefit." My personal favorite: "Use of phospholipase derived from pig pancreas would be unacceptable to vegetarians and some religious groups . . ."

All of these—thirty-odd additives including reducing agents like L-cysteine hydrochloride for stretchiness—produce a light, fluffy, uniform bread slice that balls up and sticks to the roof of your mouth, says Whitley; it can be used in an emergency to gather up minute slivers of broken glass from the floor. He understands that while low cost does not always translate to inferior quality, limited resources also limit choice. Reading his book, I was reminded that a mom or dad on a tight budget shopping for the family at a supermarket will almost certainly not buy a five- or six-dollar local artisan whole-wheat walnut bread in a nearby bin, no matter how tempting. Their issue is more likely to find the most healthful $1.99 sliced sandwich bread, which will be made from industrial wheat. Safe to eat, yes. Highly nutritional, probably not. But the word has spread sufficiently about white bread by now to create more demand for packaged whole wheat: even at 51 percent a better choice, and some large industrial manufacturers manage to produce it in that price range.

Whitley, for his part, gets past his depressing inventory of the Chorleywood's nonnatural bread components to entertain us with historical snippets. He takes us inside a famous 1860s Russian cookbook written by Elena Molokhovets in which she explains how to gauge when unbaked loaves are ready to bake. "You may put the loaves in a bucket of water (the temperature of a river in summer) where they will lie on the bottom until fully proofed. When they float to the surface put them straight in the oven."

No bobbing loaves on summer rivers floating by my kitchen windows at last sight, but I trust Whitley to guide me over any and all terrain, wet or dry. He comes across as a man who'd gladly sleep on a bed of warm Scottish Morning Rolls and climb into any bowl of fermenting dough large enough to accommodate an inquiring, respectful visitor.

Flipping to the rear of *Bread Matters*, I choose a formula for a basic multigrain sourdough, and I'm off.

The $158 Loaf

All of my environmentally aware, resource-conscious credentials seem to be in order. I've created a starter using free and available wild yeasts circulating in the fresh air around me; my organic whole-wheat flour was milled only twenty-three miles away, by Central Milling in Petaluma, California, and delivered to my local Whole Foods that I ride my bike to whenever possible to reduce my carbon footprint. The organic wheat itself was grown sustainably in the high country of Utah, not around the corner but not halfway across the country in Kansas, either. I'm reasonably sure that my Portuguese Flor de Sal was hand-harvested with energy-efficient scraping rakes by fair-trade laborers and that no sea urchins were orphaned in the process.

None of that I need mention to Bonnie, who makes an occasional appearance, taking a deep sniff or two at my request as my starter begins to bubble away. No doubt she's regretted more than once that she even brought up her glutenized neck for discussion, especially now, standing in a kitchen that she no longer recognizes as her own. Where juicers and blenders once sat whirring up kale-and-banana-and whey-and-chia-seed smoothies, bakers' items sprawl over the counter space they no longer occupy. I've done the research. Which is why we now own $158 worth of paraphernalia: a must-have baker's scale that weighs in grams as well as in ounces and pounds.

Also proofing baskets, called bannetons, for the second rise and the couches, or cotton towels that sit inside; dough whisks, a bench knife or dough cutter, a lame or scoring knife, parchment paper, a Dutch oven; cooling racks; and various recommended implements whose purpose I've yet to determine.

"Just the essentials," I assure her.

Someday perhaps I'll add an electric mixer, but that can wait. Mixing by hand, my baker friends tell me, is the only way to learn to judge the readiness of dough as your fingers become familiar over time with the exact textural feel of the stages of development.

A large glass bowl contains what Whitley calls a production sourdough and most others refer to as a pre-ferment; by any name a portion of my mature starter blended with added whole-wheat, rye, and bread (white) flour and water. It will sit covered at room temperature for sixteen hours or more, the slow fermentation ensuring that microbes and enzymes have ample time to go about their assorted processes of breaking down protein and sugar molecules. After which I hand-mix it with more flour and water and perform a variety of maneuvers, all designed to produce a crispy-crusted loaf with a silky interior, or crumb.

Hand mixing I find to be basically hiring yourself out as a physical therapist, the dough being your flabby client whose flaccid muscles become sturdy, toned, and taut only if worked hard, so five hundred times or more—"you can't mix too much," bakers advise—you scoop and stretch and massage and yank and pull until your arms ache and the dough gluten you've activated after ten to fifteen nonstop minutes finally begins to push back. At that juncture scooping becomes a full-on tussle; the battle is enjoined. As the dough's elastic sinews develop and the cool rubbery texture takes on an appealing resilience, it now clings to itself and no longer to your fingers, a gratifying reward for your strenuous efforts. Many bakers describe the process as meditative, in the same way that yoga can stress your body while relaxing your mind.

That's what should happen. My first effort doesn't quite follow standard practice. Next to me throughout is *Bread Matters*, whose "Really Simple Sourdough Bread" recipe provides my inspiration and step-by-step guidance. Over the enterprise of making sourdough breads at home, Whitley reminds me, "hangs an aura of mysticism, a sense that the processes involved may be accessible only to a chosen few. The sourdough grail is guarded by zealots, who expatiate interminably on the size of the holes in the *miches*." Balderdash! says he, drawing me in with his disdain for dough snobbery. All we need do, he assures us, is trust our sense of touch, taste, and smell, pay close visual attention, and provide optimal conditions in the form of warmth and water to advance the growth of wild airborne yeast and bacteria.

This, I think, is wheat's gift to me and to all bakers. It tests us like few if any other foods to create something golden, firmly domed, and delicious from a bowl of thick gray mush. Or not. Measuring out the final ingredients on my new Ozeri Pro Digital Kitchen Food Scale, I carefully add 175 grams of water. Within minutes, as I stir the blend, I recognize that something has gone hideously wrong. My first clue is the wet wheat paste dripping from my eyelids. The dough has puddled so loosely in its bowl that a goldfish could swim laps in it. Where is the tautness, the elasticity Whitley promises? A voice inside my head squeals like a young John McEnroe, "You *cannot* be *serious*!" Fortunately Bonnie is away from home at her office, it's mid-morning, and I'm soaked to the skin through my shirt, covered everywhere with soggy dollops of splashed, powdered, wet wheat.

Making a weak attempt to reach a dripping arm toward *Bread Matters* for further help, I spray this clotted mess over the book's opened pages, then try with an elbow to lift the handle of the sink faucet to wash off under clear running water. That more or less works, and glancing back at the book as I wipe off face and hands, an idea comes to me: Andrew Whitley is an alive person, and people exist somewhere in the flesh. Andrew Whitley can explain to me perhaps exactly what he could possibly have had in mind with these ridiculous measurements, and maybe even suggest a remedy after I finish dressing him down for the swamp I'm now paddling in.

As a journalist I've made a habit of popping into the lives of strangers without knocking first, then peppering them with questions they have no need to answer. Most do, for reasons that remain unclear. In short order I locate Whitley's phone number on his breadmatters website, learn that he now lives on a farm in Lamancha, West Linton, Scottish Borders just south of Edinburgh. I calculate the time zone difference, and as I punch his number I imagine him just sitting down to after-dinner single malt, neat, with eyes cast under his Tam o'Shanter looking out toward Loch Lomond. I hope to ruin his evening but good.

After a few rings a man picks up and asks in a plummy English baritone who might be calling. And just as quickly I lose my edge. It's the plumminess. Soothing, cushioning, bringing to mind the melodious resonance of Laurence Olivier and John Gielgud. I introduce myself and mention the wheat book I'm writing, but he's hardly fooled. "You're calling for baking help, is that it?" The desperation in my voice must hum through the line like an electrical current.

"Well, there is a bit of an issue, yes." And I briefly outline the situation as rivulets of grainy water continue to run down inside my shirt.

" 'Lumpy soup,' you said?"

"It's that sort of consistency, yup. It's not the taut rubber band you mention, where you grasp ahold of the kneaded dough and stretch it before your eyes until you can see through its center."

"Hmmm."

"It's not—" and at that moment, wiping muck off the Ozeri scale beside me, I inadvertently turn it back on and glance down to the unit measurement options barely visible in mouse type along the right border in contrast to the large bold numeric display digits. Mine is set for "oz"—ounces, not "gm," for grams, the unit I intended to program, following his instructions.

"Is everything all right, then?" Andrew must have heard me gasp. I realize in an instant that since there are twenty-eight grams to an ounce, by miscalculation I've added twenty-eight times more water to my mix than the recipe calls for, closer to a gallon than the recommended three-quarter cup. I suddenly see myself starring in a lost episode of *I Love Lucy*, the one where Lucy and I stand drenched to our waists in flour broth as the kitchen floods and Fred Mertz walks in, surveys the scene, and comments out of the side of his mouth, "Well, why don't we all get into our bathing suits and whip up a few more loaves?"

I don't know how to convey this to Whitley without sounding anything less than moronic. "Oh, wait, I may have found the glitch," I mutter at a barely audible level into the phone. No fool, he clearly gets that it's operator error, and nothing but.

"Well, good then." Whitley is wrapping up his end of it. Yet another hapless Yankee. I come back to my senses just in time to steer the subject to his lifelong passion for wheat, rye, and other whole grains. What motivated it? I ask, mopping up. "Bread baking has allowed me to exercise my manual and intellectual side, both the Tolstoy and Chekhov in me that are usually at war, and to do so in perfect harmony, which I accept as a rare gift." That's how Whitley talks, with an effortless literary cadence that most writers strive for in vain. His life's work, he adds, has been to deliver the full nutritional value of whole grains in baked goods that people are eager to consume.

Going with the Grain

The subject of a healthful loaf is politically charged for Whitley. Everybody, he says, should be within walking distance of real bread. "The way in which the majority of bread now is made may well have facets which validate the anti-wheat thesis. Raw materials play a role but 75 to 80 percent is in the process. If it's not long-fermented sixteen hours or more, if it's sped through as instant dough, the industrial method, it simply won't make the kernel's nutrients available to the body They go straight through to the sewer. It can also cause digestive issues, especially for gluten-sensitives."

By now we've been chatting for close to an hour. Springing from topic to topic, the conversation keeps circling back to his devotion to whole-grain, rye, and wheat sourdoughs and his conviction that technological advances in production have improved efficiency and volume at the expense of nutrition and flavor. These deficiencies in modern wheat, he argues—as do many others—directly result from fifty years of breeding to create varieties that thrive on heavy feedings of soluble fertilizers, especially nitrogen, to increase yield.

By Whitley's account the hollow straw stalks in turn become more susceptible to fungal and pest attacks. Shorter stem length and tighter seed heads bred to boost endosperm content for bread making, another breakthrough, create smaller canopies that expose the soil to more weed growth, entailing increased herbicide and pesticide use. Nutritional value gets such short shrift in all this, he adds, that it rarely enters into consideration.

Whitley's passion for sourdough—his new recipe book devoted to it, *Do Sourdough: Slow Bread for Busy Lives*, came out in 2014—inspired me to dust myself off and start again. I didn't know at the time that over the next year or so I would fall madly, deeply, truly in love with the microbial universe of long-fermented wheat and the crunchy, tangy, chewy morsels of baked breads it spawned. Bonnie began to suspect something was up when she caught me refreshing my sourdough starter at four in the morning, crooning to it like a newborn. I listened with glee as it emitted little burps of carbon dioxide gas—for my ears only—on its way to leavening my loaves. I soon noticed that I was timing my writing breaks to coincide with the hourly schedule for folding bulk-fermented dough by hand as part of the bread-making process. A semipermanent film of wheat flour bonded to every surface in our kitchen. To me it was not schmutz, it was a diaphanous bride's veil.

Looking on as I consumed slices of my own sourdough every day, eating more bread in one week than in two months before any of this began, Bonnie suggested that I might want to audition as the cover boy for the next edition of *Wheat Belly*. Instead I began to drop pounds while making no other changes in my exercise routine or food selections. That weight loss, you better believe, caught my wife's attention. By now, about four months into her gluten-free, mirth-free dieting, she reported that the initial clarity and energy boost had leveled off some. I noted that on occasion she eyed my linen-wrapped loaves with more than casual interest, but I made no attempt to persuade her to sample the bread—although that took some restraint. Inside every journalist is an evangelist struggling to get out.

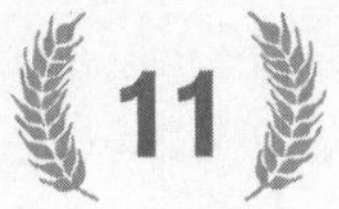

Ancient Wisdom

> Convince me that you have a seed there, and I am prepared to expect wonders.
>
> —Henry David Thoreau

When a wheat spike matures into a head, it produces somewhere between twenty and fifty kernels tucked inside its vertical argyle pattern of golden fiber strands that dance in perfect rhythmic unison with thousands of others under a summer breeze. A flowing field of wind-tossed wheat stalks may inspire poetry and song, but not hunger: the last thing you'd guess is that any part of the bristly thatched shoot is edible.

We did, as a species. We figured that out, possibly out of desperation, and went about inventing myriad involved methods of breeding and growing its kernels, processing them, and turning that discovery to our own advantage. An evolutionary leap, or so I thought until I came across the perspective of another renegade thinker like Whitley—the author of the provocative *Guns, Germs, and Steel*, Jared Diamond. He takes a jaundiced view of that transition, staking out a position so boldly out of synch with conventional wisdom that it deserves an airing before moving along.

To me, our segue from spear-thrower to seed planter constituted an epic advance for mankind. I reasoned that as enticing as the Paleolithic diet may be to many, we can enjoy those foods at home because we have a permanent, stationary living space—that is, a home—to shelter us as we sit down to eat. That concept derived from the advent of agriculture, from which sprang communities that spawned villages, then cities and all of the political, cultural, and social institutions that intersect with our lives today. I took that to be the logical and laudable progression until I came upon Diamond's essay, "The Worst Mistake in the History of the Human Race." He argues the opposite point of view. "Recent discoveries suggest that the adoption of agriculture, supposedly our most decisive step toward a better life, was in many ways a catastrophe from which we have never recovered. With agriculture came the gross social and sexual inequality, the disease and despotism, that curse our existence." Wheat was foremost among the eight "founder crops" that doomed us.

Diamond accepts that while for many hunter-gatherers life might have been nasty, brutish, and short, it was also sustained by eating wild animals and wild plants, foods that "provide more protein and a better balance of other nutrients." By contrast, "today just three high-carbohydrate plants—wheat, rice, and corn—provide the bulk of the calories consumed by the human species, yet each one is deficient in certain vitamins or amino acids essential to life."

In her *New Yorker* overview of the current Paleolithic trend, Elizabeth Kolbert points to research that indicates that the transition from hunting to plowing was, in its own way, equally brutish. A study of human remains in China and Japan reveals that the average person's height declined by three inches with the advent of rice cultivation; a similar decline occurred as wheat spread from the Middle

East across Europe. Deadly epidemics increased as people began living closer together, creating societies that were ideal breeding grounds for microbes.

At the very least, these writers made me reconsider the meaning of *progress*. In balance, I'm still persuaded that more good than harm came from our adoption of agriculture. Yet I also know that an astonishing one third of our population—over a hundred million Americans—are obese at present, and that refined grains act as a mainline injection system for starch. In refined flour nothing slows the breakdown of starch to glucose, which travels directly through the porous intestinal wall into the bloodstream. Considering the prevalence today of diabetes and other glucose-related conditions, I do wonder at times if self-inflicted illness will go down as one of the unintended by-products of our hunter-to-planter transition. "We're still struggling with the mess into which agriculture has tumbled us," Diamond concludes, "and it's unclear whether we can solve it."

Natural Identity

Diamond may be denouncing all agriculture anywhere, but, even so, I think I may have given him reason to reconsider if I'd taken him with me on my excursion to meet one of Northern California's most informed sustainable wheat growers and produce farmers, Paul Muller. For reasons that were self-serving as well as research-oriented, I decided to follow one of Community Grains' wheats back to its source—the "Identity Preserved" Durum Iraq from Full Belly Farm. I'd been spending way too much time inside, an occupational hazard of the writing life, and I needed a hit of manure, dirt, hay, and compost. I've been growing organic vegetables for decades, and I'm so committed to the therapeutic healing value of turning soil and starting seeds that I'm convinced all psychiatrists should dump the couch, replace it with a planter box, and hand out pitchforks to everyone who enters their office. Neuroses don't stand a chance against the heart's joy in nurturing that fertile speck of nothing into a sugar snap pea pod.

More to the point, I wanted to investigate the heritage and heirloom varieties now being revived from Washington to California on one coast and from Maine to Anson Mills in South Carolina on the Eastern Seaboard. (I use *heritage* and *heirloom* interchangeably to refer to seeds that have been saved and passed down for at least fifty years, often for a hundred or more. After 1945 industrial improvements in agriculture gave rise to the vast expansion of single or monoculture American non-heirlooms that rely on inorganic chemicals.)

And while we're at it, in the parlance of the grain and soybean industries, *identity-preserved* (better known as IP) refers to specialty, high-value, premium, or niche market products, while commodity grains are marketed in mass, often as livestock feed. An IP wheat variety might cover only 60,000 of 8.4 million acres planted in Kansas, or less than 100 at a small organic farm like Full Belly, where six active partners including Paul Muller and Dru Rivers, and three of their four grown children, raise all manner of crops including Durum Iraq and Frassinetto, an Italian landrace, or locally grown heirloom dating back to 1927, with up to 13 percent protein level.

Wheat grows among a bountiful diversity of vegetables, herbs, nuts, and fruits that includes almonds, pomegranates, basil, peaches, and figs, 450 acres in all, tended to by about sixty employees and home to a herd of sheep, a tribe of goats, a flock of chickens, and a few cows. Located in Guinda in the fertile Capay Valley of Yolo County, California, Full Belly puts Muller's theories about sustainable farming to the test, especially in a drought year like 2014 when his crops received only one third of the normal rainfall, following an even drier previous year. Scanning other fields on the way to his farm, I passed row after row of shriveled, parched, young wheat.

When you drive down a long dirt road to enter the Full Belly compound, you come upon a small community complete with toddlers, dogs, redwood barns and storage buildings, farming equipment and assorted dust-layered vehicles, also bins of newly harvested flowers, vegetables, and fruit. Country casual overlays organized productivity; some teams clean, store, and ready harvested crops for wholesale and farmer's market and CSA (community-supported agriculture) farm box-to-consumer delivery while others prepare food for the crews and keep an eye on the youngsters. I arrived just before lunchtime, my good luck. Within a few minutes I was eating Dru's homemade bread and dill-laced beet soup and fresh-picked salad while the grandson of Paul and Dru crawled between my feet at a long picnic table. "I love growing wheat," Muller was telling me, "the real thing, as you'll see. Can it thrive using an organic system? That's what we're checking out. Borlaug created his high-yield mutant for good reasons, but he mutated a crop that's been evolving with us for ten thousand years, with our own enzymes and gut bacteria."

The essence of Muller's approach as he sees it is working with the rhythms of nature, not in a combative mode. To that end he intersperses flowers for bee pollination with vegetable crops to invite and nourish beneficial insects. Others gate-crash, too. When we arrived at his two wheat plantings after lunch, both green and flourishing in early spring, I saw at once how alive the stalks and budding heads were with foraging critters. "You're looking at lygus bugs and the twelve-spotted cucumber beetle," he told me as we bent close. "Lygus can puncture a plant's outer glume and suck up sap, not good, so what we do is give them something to chew on. We plant yarrow with those neighboring strawberries over there."

Mule Farmers

What impressed Muller most about his wheat was its bright green vigor. "We're still in the middle of March and all around us, up and down the valley, wheat fields are already browning." He attributed the vitality of his plants to a good cover crop that harnessed and preserved moisture, and to the microbial healthfulness of the soil. "There are *billions* of microbes in every few inches of that soil, we've now learned. That's our main job, to manage the microbiome. It takes time, as it should."

Chemical farming, in Muller's view, is racehorse farming—high inputs like inorganic nitrogen produce high-yield fast results but deliver no character. "We're mule farmers by comparison." As he scans the two adjacent wheat fields, he gestures with a sweep of his hand. "But look at how different one is from the other." He's read my mind. The Iraq is hearty, with fat heads. The Frassinetto is more anemic by comparison: narrow heads, a paler green. "Those Italian seeds may be pinched when we harvest in June or July. But hopefully they'll get to the end of their cycle in shape to be milled."

Klein, who is buying both varieties for Community Grains, used Certified to mill Full Belly's harvested kernels. A few years back, when Muller brought in his first Iraq crop, it registered only 11 percent protein, way below average for durum.

"Don't waste your money," Vanderliet told them both. "You'll never get good pasta out of that."

I could easily imagine the steely-eyed certainty with which Joe V delivered that verdict, and also the dejection that would normally follow from grower and buyer. But Muller and Klein didn't buckle under. "We want it milled anyway," they said. Joe V obliged. Klein's crew extruded the pasta from the semolina in the kitchen at Oliveto and discovered it to be, in Klein's words, "the best we ever tasted! Nutty. Rich. Silky firm. Totally wonderful." For Klein, that success confirmed the possibility of bringing off his dream of a functioning local grain economy that delivered superior products.

Looking back, Muller explains that there was no market incentive at first, half a decade ago, to grow heritage wheat. No one paid attention to flavor. "Then with Bob and a few others showing up, flavor and whole-grain integrity took on value, at least to the extent we could grow the wheat and break even. You make just about enough farming sustainably and organically to keep going because it's so labor intensive."

Farmer's markets, CSAs, retail, and wholesale outlets like Whole Foods provide the income for Full Belly. At sixty-one, with four grown children in all, one still in college and the others working onsite, Muller gets up in the morning and his hands have plunged deep into the soil somewhere on his acreage before breakfast. By his choice, and Dru's, their farm has also become an educational center for sustainable organic agriculture. They see themselves as stewards of the land, passing along to the next generation a philosophy that encompasses vibrant food, stable employment, and a commitment to local food systems. There are no gluten necks anywhere in sight, or *Wheat Belly* cage rattlers.

"We live in paradise," Muller tells me as I'm about to depart. "All you have to do is pay attention and not screw it up."

Living Flour

On the opposite coast in Columbia, South Carolina, at Anson Mills, Glenn Roberts, when not growing and milling Carolina Gold rice, devotes himself and his resources to growing heirloom varieties of wheat on his own farms and with partnering farmers. "When I go out into a field of heirloom wheat, Red Fife or Sonora White or Farro Piccolo [einkorn], I nibble on the berries, you have to, to know when it's time to cut it; you can't go out there with a moisture meter, it doesn't do you any good, so when you speak about culinary enjoyment I'd *pay* to do that, berry-chew, the flavors are *beyond* understanding!" Roberts talks in torrents, a gushing flood that saturates you with his encyclopedic knowledge of all things granular, swept along by currents of passion. Once you adjust to the speed and volume, abundant nuggets of historical details, anecdotes, and opinions wash up to be gleaned. Before industrialization, he says, wheats weren't just "nutty" or "rich," they delivered vanilla-cream and honeysuckle and a whole spice rack of delicious flavors. "That's what I look for, terroir. I've taken to hand-threshing in the field, truly by hand, not even with a scythe, milling a sample by rubbing it hard between my palms and sometimes fermenting it in the field. There's a whole brothy, aley thing you get, too, and minerality."

To preserve the nutrients and intense flavors of the wheats he harvests, Roberts, whose mother, a gifted pastry chef, served her family only desserts for dinner on Sundays as a special treat, developed his own stone-milling methods. "As much as I love pastry, and the elastic thinking of pastry chefs to this day—I married one—have I become an advocate of refined white flour? No! But I'm an advocate of alive bolted flour." (Bolting lightens whole-wheat flour by sifting out the larger bran shards without depleting its fiber, nutrients, or minerals.) Things get complicated quickly in Roberts's telling because that "alive" flour contains germ oils that go rancid in a flash. To circumvent the problem, Roberts says, "We marry the high and the low, the old and the new. We're stone-milling but not in any way that anyone would recognize. We're milling at minus ten degrees Fahrenheit, fresh to order, there's no milling cycle over five minutes from wheat berry to package, all under a carbon dioxide envelope from the freezer."

Oxygenation quickly come into play. "We don't want these things to go dormant, so we keep CO_2 in there, which forces the berries to reach for oxygen and keep them aerobic. Why? Nobody talks about the viability of aerobic cultures in live flours, even though in preindustrial days they would be milling aerobic wheat right into the ferment, with the vat next to the plant. That's how we mill. There are a lot of chefs cold-milling now, which is great, but no one like us in the States. In Europe, maybe, there's a long tradition from antiquity of milling in the dead of winter."

Anson grows and mills primarily for chefs, but also sells milled Red Fife and Red May, America's first farmer-selected production wheat, direct to customers on its website along with antebellum grits—"the best anywhere," a friend told me—and cornmeal, polenta, coarse Graham wheat flour, Abruzzi heirloom rye flour, farro, and more. The site also reflects Roberts's historical grasp of the connection between the health of grain and the prosperity of the civilization growing it. Since antiquity, he reports, artisan loaves have always been crafted from exceptional wheat, available solely when the society farming it was on a rise or near apogee. As a result, not only are you able to gauge the economic and social status of citizens in any Western culture down the millennia by the color of the bread they were eating, but the economic standing of the city, state, or nation, too, by the relative abundance of artisan breads.

I came for insights into artisan wheat farming and will leave Roberts's company with a trove of lore including specific wheat varieties introduced to the South by Huguenots, Germans, Sephardim, and the Italians, who brought farro to Carolina's rice fields just before the start of the eighteenth century. Brewsters, Celtic grain women in the British Isles, grew numerous individual wheat varieties in a single field centuries ago, I learn, then selected out their preferences. Transposed to our shores by American colonists, that tradition survived until the invention of the roller mill—and has begun to be successfully resurrected by artisan growers-slash-millers like indefatigable Roberts.

If We Build It . . .

In keeping with his agenda to support and improve lands through sustainable farming practices—growing grains, legumes, and brassicas in rotation—last summer Roberts flew to Southern California to fund and provide seeds for the Common Grain project. Initiated by Japanese chef, food writer, and teacher Sonoko Sakai in Los Angeles, her "grain hub" unites growers, millers, and bakers to produce items made with heirloom and ancient grains. A prominent cookbook author and chef, Sakai makes and teaches the art of creating fresh, exquisitely buoyant, and flavorful soba and udon, among other Asian specialties including rice balls. She's so devoted to using nothing but properly stone-milled flour that she brings suitcases of finely ground buckwheat back to Los Angeles from the only source she trusts in Japan. But she tells me that sustaining live soil to produce many different varieties of live flour is a special passion, and nothing excites her like grain, because she knows what you can do with it if you know what you're doing.

Ironically, up to 90 percent of soft white wheat, from eastern Washington's Palouse area, is exported to Asia, and Japan buys up to 96 percent of all the buckwheat (no genetic relation to wheat) grown in the United States. Sonoko Sakai says she travels to Japan to load up on grain grown in America, a wearying transpacific crisscross she hopes to eliminate one day by starting her own customized noodle-flour stone mill in California or Washington.

With her seed grant from Anson Mills, she enlisted farmers in Santa Barbara and Kern Counties to grow emmer, Sonora, and Red Fife heirlooms. Soft-white Sonora came up through Mexico in the 1700s, while hard Red Fife came down from Canada about a century later. "Local artisan bakers led me to the potential growers who were supplying restaurants with organic heirloom produce, like tomatoes. They'd never heard of a similar category of wheat, but when they checked they found Glenn's heirlooms to be an ideal rotation crop for their soil."

Roberts, who goes about the country dispensing his trove to local grain growers like a Johnny Wheatseed, joins a dedicated, loosely organized coalition of locally grown and freshly stone-milled ancient and heritage grain producers that includes Klein's Community Grains and Monica Spiller's Whole Grain Connection in Northern California; the Hayden Flour Mill in Tempe, Arizona; the Maine Grain Alliance, Grist and Toll in Pasadena; Thom Leonard's Heartland Mill in Marienthal, Kansas; the Washington State growers and millers in Skagit Valley, as well as a burgeoning local grain movement in New York and Massachusetts.

Their prevailing ethos, "If we build it, they will come," may gain traction in future years, but at the moment the assumptions behind that rousing declamation still tilt toward wishful thinking. Full disclosure: as a website content director I was deeply involved in the dot-com bubble burst a decade or so back, where an identical "Field of Dreams" mantra ended with hundreds of start-ups including Webvan and Pets.com blowing through enormous sums of money before evaporating overnight. The only folks who showed up in the end were creditors and burned investors.

So, based on past experience I may not be the most objective observer, but even with the best of intentions local grain faces formidable obstacles: educating the public, turning a profit, and building an efficient infrastructure stand out as three of the most daunting, especially at a time when the media and consumers are not exactly embracing wheat with open arms. I expect that if successful, the strongest selling points for fresh local whole-wheat flour and baked goods will be vivid, pure flavor, as found in organic carrots and organic tomatoes, and nutritional benefits that matter and do not compromise eating pleasure. They're real enough, but nobody's figured out how to make them the leading factor in driving sales. "To me whole grains are the single most important indicator of overall health," University of Minnesota public health professor David Jacobs told the Community Grains Conference.

That, I thought to myself at the time, could up the ante as long as artisans are able to counter the conventional wisdom that whole wheat is a granular version of castor oil and needs to be adulterated with sweeteners to make it palatable. Jacobs proceeds with the restraint of a seasoned academic researcher and mathematical statistician wedded to the factual analysis of patterns. As an epidemiologist he looks at how often, where, and why diseases appear, or don't, in various groups of people. "Most of the many substances in the bran and the germ are foreign to the human body, but much evidence suggests that these substances are important for human health," he wrote in an e-mail after the conference. Jacobs specializes in food synergy, a subject he's explored in numerous papers.

When we followed up with a phone conversation, he defined food synergy as the complex interactions of thousands of compounds involved in the digestive process. In his view, stripping out and reinserting nutrients is likely to compromise those processes. "I'm skeptical about simplistic explanations when talking about gliadin and gluten, and broad statements that wheat is bad, whole or refined. What we've found over twenty years of tracking diets and their connection to diseases is that populations that eat more whole grains are less likely to succumb to fatal diseases."

In an oft-cited Iowa Women's Health Study, Jacobs and his team reported that women who ate two or more servings of whole grains a day were 30 percent less likely to have died from an inflammation-related condition. "People who eat that way simply have a lower mortality rate in study after study." His findings were amplified by a Harvard Public Health study released in early 2015, which found that whole grains extended life spans by 10 percent for 110,000 men and women followed over two decades.

Jacobs went on to tell me that whole-grain eaters tend to be nonsmokers who are thinner and more physically active. "They come with a constellation of healthy lifestyle habits."

Wheat Belly's author, I reminded him, claims that the difference between eating whole and white-flour wheat is the difference between smoking filtered and non-filtered cigarettes: both kill you. Jacobs batted away Davis's hypothesis without pause. "If you do the statistical techniques to break out whole grain, you find it is predictive of reduced chronic disease rates. That, too, is very consistent." The studies, he added, point in one direction: "Whole grains and seeds are very good for you."

Ancient Future

Taking stock of Jacobs's comments, delivered in an unwavering monotone, I noted that they gain a degree of credibility by the total absence of emotion he attaches to them. Diets in general and gluten in particular tap into a reservoir of impassioned advocacy, and the intensity of the heat often obscures the suspicious origins of the fire. More than ever before, we're seeking advice on how best to serve the needs of our bodies and brains while being asked to sort through ever-increasing mounds of conflicting data. That presents an ideal environment for dogmatic evangelists to step up and oversell their simplistic gospels.

If weight loss alone and nothing else mattered and all flour, whole or refined, added unwanted pounds, we could simply stop eating it. But 100 percent whole-grain wheat, as Jacobs and hundreds of other researchers have asserted for decades, arrives with a long list of nourishing, immune system–enhancing attributes from minerals to vitamins to fiber that even the most nutritious non-gluten substitutes like quinoa, with 65 percent less fiber, do not replicate as a complete package. And it now develops that the friendliest bacteria in our gut feed off fiber, adding to whole wheat's attributes.

The best of both worlds, ironically, may exist in ancient varieties—emmer, einkorn, spelt, and khorasan, trademarked as Kamut—a class of whole wheats promoted by some local economy grain crusaders that seems to be better tolerated by many with gluten sensitivity. In spite of their differing gliadin-to-glutenin ratios, these wheats are sufficiently strong in overall protein to allow leavened dough to bake without collapsing in the oven. Celiac disease sufferers, however, cannot safely consume any of these.

I at first categorized ancient-grainers as the fringe element of a niche movement, the sect within the cult. For millers and professional bakers, ancestral wheat flours present a unique set of challenges. As hulled wheats (excluding Kamut), the tough glume enclosure does not break free from the grain, so they require slower and more costly processing; for bakers, they respond to hydration and yeast differently from bread wheat; and for most home bread bakers, they usually require a trip to gourmet shops or health food stores, or a visit to the few specialty grain online sources; scarcity and extra labor boost the retail price of ancient varieties to double or triple standard flour.

But funny things happen, even to wheat. Early in 2014 celebrity chef and baker Chad Robertson published his third cookbook, *Tartine Book No. 3: Modern Ancient Classic Whole*, and ancient got hip overnight. Famed for his silky, crunchy French country loaves, Robertson and Tartine had already developed a wide national following, and now he had a great story to tell to admiring fans about how he and his wife, pastry chef Liz Prueitt, discovered and experimented with wheats from antiquity to turn out flavor-bursting sweet and savory baked gems. With the same disarming mix of restless curiosity and boyish enthusiasm that won over *Martha Stewart* audiences and social media acolytes (male-model handsome helps, too), Robertson extolled the virtues of wheat-spelt crispbreads, chamomile-Kamut shortbread, buckwheat-hazelnut sables, and dozens of other what-the-hell-is-this-anyway pastries, porridge breads, and ancient grain creations such as spelt and toasted corn-flour baguettes. Your odds of making these at home or chancing upon them at your local bakery may be minimal to nonexistent, but to Robertson the recipes confirmed his commitment to inspire, provoke, and expand the art and science of his chosen craft.

By my reckoning, Robertson is exactly what the local grain economy needs and, more specifically, the heritage and ancient varieties it promotes. He makes wheat sexy and enticing, feelings that are difficult to muster watching a massive mechanical combine mow down half the state of Kansas.

Many of the new Tartine cookbook's recipes come from Scandinavia, Germany, and Austria, countries where Robertson and his wife and business partner, Liz, explored baking traditions; some are from France, where Robertson first learned to bake, working with spelt in Provence. There's a romantic yarn to be told about harvesting that rare wheat in the mountains as an apprentice and, once home, adopting the techniques of ancient wheat growers like the Dane Claus Meyer to what Robertson calls "the California idiom." In the book's foreword he writes eloquently about looking to the past while pushing ahead. "It is, in some sense, a journey backward, an attempt to . . . rejoin our nascent age of invention." Ancient wheats, he contends, combine delicate gluten with higher protein, making them easier to digest, especially when long-fermented with a natural leaven.

Where all this leads remains open to debate. Nothing without gluten that calls itself bread at present satisfies the visceral, deep-seeded (in every sense) crunchy-silky wheat craving that galvanizes bread lovers. Ancient wheats seem to provide a partial, if not entirely satisfying solution. Scientific studies posted by the Whole Grains Council on its informative website indicate that diploid einkorn with a meager fourteen chromosomes compared to modern bread wheat's forty-two, along with durum (twenty-eight chromosomes), is comfortably tolerated by many gluten-sensitive individuals.

Saving Julia

Eager to learn more about that, I contacted Carla Bartolucci. She and her husband, Rodolfo, founded Jovial Foods, one of the very few American companies growing, manufacturing, and selling einkorn. Up to 20 percent higher in protein, einkorn, like all wheats, lacks sufficient lysine to form a complete protein source while delivering more potassium, phosphorus, iron, and magnesium than modern wheat. On Jovial's website, a graph shows the ancient grain to contain 15 percent less starch than commercial bread wheat, along with beta-carotene lutein, a powerful antioxidant associated with eye health, and also a larger volume of vitamin E. I knew just enough about einkorn, itself genetically unchanged over ten thousand years, to admire its flavor and wonder about the motivation of anyone willing to take on the obstacles required to bring a specialty grain to market. I had already bought a few pounds of Jovial's einkorn flour and made my own loaf of sourdough; starting off as a sticky dough, it surprised me with its light, pliable crust, its abundant small air holes, its sweet nuttiness, and its inviting scent of custard in the soft yellow crumb—not at all what I was expecting from a Neolithic grass that my Stone Age ancestors pounded into porridge.

Carla first explained why she and Rudolfo, with connections to Italian organic farmers through a previous business, became interested in einkorn. "Our daughter, Julia, then seven and now fourteen, was really an unhealthy kid. She had gastroenteritis, then after that constant diarrhea, and she even began to lose her hair. Our pediatrician thought the problem was lactose intolerance, but when that didn't help we took her off eggs and tried everything including a gluten-free diet. But I didn't want to pursue gluten-free if I didn't have to because it meant eating a lot of bad starches. By then we'd moved back to Italy, to Modena, and a homeopathic doctor suggested that maybe Julia could tolerate ancient wheat. We tried spelt and Kamut but they didn't improve her situation. So we asked around to researchers, what is really the most ancient wheat? One led us to einkorn."

It was the Bartoluccis' good fortune that a dozen years earlier the intact body of Ötzi the Iceman had been discovered high up in the Alps, and that just before he was clubbed to death in 3300 BCE, the last meal he'd eaten consisted of wild goat meat and bread made from einkorn. That prompted a flurry of scientific research on the grain in Italy, among other countries, creating an archive of information accumulated over twelve years. Commercial availability lagged behind—and that gave the couple an idea: why not try to produce it commercially as well to share its benefits.

"We actually found a farmer in our town who agreed to plant the seeds we obtained through the research association, about fifty test acres," Carla told me. "Once we grew it and milled it, we started Julia on an einkorn diet. Her asthma had gotten much worse, surprisingly, since we'd moved to Modena. Her nose was completely plugged; she had intestinal issues, skin rashes, enlarged tonsils, dark bags under her eyes, and she also could get very, very moody. By nature she's a bright, wonderful, positive person, but at times she could be really unbearable. Very strange. But when we took everything wheat-based except einkorn out of her diet, after about two months the symptoms really cleared up. A year passed before the lining of her intestines completely healed, and by then her hair had started growing back in a crown, with bangs! It was incredible, the transformation."

Based on her daughter's recovery, Carla and Rudolfo enlisted the help of Italian farmers with small organic acreage and convinced them to plant a seed they'd never come across, then contracted with a specialty mill set up to process hulled wheats, since emmer—as farro—and spelt are both popular in Italy.

"The difference between einkorn and regular wheat is not that it is lower in gluten," she said. "It has the same amount or more, but the gluten is completely different. Einkorn does not contain the high molecular proteins that are in all other types of wheat and that many people have a hard time digesting. It's very weak gluten, and for that reason, easier to digest." Geneticist Bob Graybosch, for one, takes issue with Bartolucci. "I can find plenty of papers describing high-molecular weight glutenins in einkorn wheat," he told me. He also questioned any link between gluten strength and digestibility. "When the acids and enzymes in our gut hit them, does it make any difference how strong they are in the baking process?"

I asked her to send me confirming research and scouted around on my own. A chapter on einkorn in a scientific anthology on flour and bread quotes two studies that "suggest a reduced or absent toxicity of *T. monococcum* [einkorn] which lacks a highly immunoreactive gliadin." This ancient grain, in other words, appears to be safer. Other studies report that einkorn contains less sugar-spiking amylopectin starch and more slow-releasing amylose, all to the good. Having burrowed as a nonscientist into mounds of research papers since delving into the wheat-gluten hullabaloo, I've learned to approach them with an equal measure of interest and wariness. A host of factors come into play, including the size of the study, the relative stature of the journal publishing it within the scientific community, and the potential impact of unacknowledged prejudices. The research team may be under pressure to achieve a specific result or confirm a bias. You and I are most likely not in a position to make a life-altering decision based on what we take away.

Carla, aware that in Italy pressures from research funders often hold sway over study results, trusted above all else her own experience with einkorn. At the same time, based on Julia's recovery and the Bartoluccis' passion for introducing others to new, quite possibly unfamiliar alternatives like einkorn, Jovial Foods was created. Today its website products include einkorn pasta and cookies as well as flour, also wheat berries, flour, a grain mill, and assorted Italian imports. Carla also teaches einkorn and gluten-free cooking classes at a villa in Lucca.

12

Taking a Stand

> The breath of the wheat and the sweet clover passed him like pleasant things in a dream.
>
> —Willa Cather, *Oh, Pioneers!*

About fifteen years ago, hiking the hills of Galilee north of Jerusalem, Eli Rogosa came across a seeded grass that the director of the Israeli gene bank identified as wild wheat. She'd found a native plant that had been growing in that area for at least five thousand years, by the gene bank director's estimate. He explained to her that it was einkorn, and with his help she was able to locate local bread made from it. For years, Rogosa told me, modern dwarf wheat had caused her to suffer miserably. But that first experience—eating the ancient wheat and discovering that, in her words, all symptoms vanished—caused her to embark on a journey to create a solution for herself and others afflicted with similar problems.

Today, as director of the Heritage Grain Conservancy in western Massachusetts, Rogosa grows einkorn and other wheats with exotic names like Zyta, Rouge de Bordeaux, and Ethiopian Purple on her twelve-acre farm, all of them organic landraces that express the unique qualities of specific environments. Paradoxically, they are genetically coded to grow and prosper in a vast range of climactic and topographical conditions as an alternative to modern hybrids dependent on the extensive, unsustainable use of fertilizers, pesticides, and irrigation. Rogosa now cultivates over one thousand wheat samples from Europe, Asia, and the Mideast that she evaluates on her farm for performance. They have to demonstrate their resilience over five years of testing before she will release them. "There will be seven billion people on earth by the next generation, and who knows what weather conditions they'll face," she says. "It's up to us to ensure that they'll have access to ancient gene pools because those wheats have endured, they've proven their capacity to survive over thousands of years. We have the power to feed ourselves as the industrial food system is struggling."

Standing Up for Bread

One thing I was sure about: while ancient and heritage grains might appeal to a broader group with time and provide a legitimate alternative to many with gluten sensitivities, they weren't likely within a foreseeable future to become readily acquirable to mainstream American consumers. I would have bet my Babe Ruth–autographed baseball bat on that, and I would have lost it to a guy whose e-mail salutation reads "Bake Like a Mutha!" He's Tom Gumpel, head baker at Panera Bread, the chain headquartered in St. Louis with close to two thousand bakery-cafés across forty-five states and Canada. By any measure it falls into the category of a mainstream middle-class enterprise, and proud of it. Panera goes through about 150 million pounds of domestic wheat a year, racks up $3 billion in annual sales, give or take a few million, and, as I quickly learned, proudly plays by its own rules. If not, Gumpel wouldn't be calling the shots. "I see our future as the go-to place for whole, ancient, and sprouted grains," he told me. "When you think of any of these as breads, or as a side with soups or salads, you will think Panera, it will make sense to you. Aspirationally that's what we're working toward."

What Gumpel has learned the hard way, he added, is that "you can't shove loaves of unfamiliar bread down the American public's throats. You deliver it in a form they're used to, like sandwich bread, the carrier, and you make that carrier a new part of the dining experience."

In mid-2014 the company banished artificial sweeteners, additives, and preservatives from its breads and everything else it serves. Gumpel, now fifty, wants to keep moving in new directions. One of ten children raised in Westchester County, and the son of a cardiologist and a nurse who moved from the Bronx when he was young, Gumpel has been in baking most of his professional life. As an eight-year-old, two of his older sisters used to take him with them to health food stores, where he discovered sprouted grains in an old refrigerator at the back of the store. One of his goals at Panera has been to drag them to the front and make them a star. The former captain of the US Baking Team that captured the grand prize at the prestigious Coupe du Monde de la Boulangerie (World Cup of Baking) in Paris, Culinary Institute of America dean, and a chef frequently listed as one the country's top ten bread bakers by industry media, Gumpel can call upon his position, prestige, and credentials to steer Panera's production to his favorite methods, souring and sprouting, and to combine them with favorite grains that rarely get an airing.

"I work with khorasan a lot, usually in a blend, not as a whole loaf. That ancient grain with its active enzymes adds a dimension of its own. It's part of our whole-grain approach."

Gumpel knows more than he ever wanted to about the wheat backlash—Panera's sales have taken a hit—and some of that rejection in his view, based on quality alone, is justified. "I pulled a slice out of the bread basket last night at a sports bar with my daughter. I wasn't thinking. I bit into it and *spit it out*! That was fast-moving yeast that didn't have an opportunity to do any work on the bread, and I'm sitting there with a mouthful of wet flour."

Panera won't play defense, even so. "This year, our slogan will be, Stand Up for Bread! We're championing a renaissance in this country. Whole and ancient grains will help us stick a fork in the ground."

The move strikes me as a bold one, a loud raspberry blown at the anti-gluten contingent whose attacks, to Gumpel, are filled with "way too many distortions."

Which put me in mind of a large sign I saw swaying above the entrance gate of the annual Kneading Conference West in Washington's Skagit Valley, north of Seattle, when I attended the gathering a few months earlier in the year. It read: LIVE FREE. EAT GLUTEN.

Tom Gumpel would have felt right at home.

Wheat-In

Until I participated in that four-day event, a collection of about 250 breadheads from twenty to eighty-plus, from professional baker to farmer to wood-fired oven builder to miller to pastry chef to avid amateur, I'd been searching in vain for a common quest that united these participants and local grain advocates everywhere, and there it was, in two words: LIVE FREE. I mulled over the phrase at length and realized it was an invitation, not a command. It invited us to disengage from the tyrannical fear that something dangerous and harmful and insidious was attacking us silently from within, throwing our systems out of harmony, depositing ugly fat on our frames, disrupting brain patterns, promoting early senility and diabetes.

As I wandered around the Research and Extension Center at Mount Vernon grounds laid out beside those fields of forty thousand experimental wheats, chatting with folks and sitting in on classes, there were moments when I thought I heard the silken sounds of Joni Mitchell's *Blue Album* wafting through the trees. This Wheat-In, a granular update of a sixties Be-In, lacked only the hookahs, patchouli, drooping pirate mustaches, swirling Indian block-print skirts, love beads, tie-dyes, and rainbow-embroidered jeans of those times long gone. There were no wheat bellies in sight, I noticed, and no demonstrations of rebellious defiance, just a bunch of people who struck me as being entirely happy in their own bodies. The expression "trust your gut" took on a new dimension of meaning for me.

In this context true wheat, "true" in the sense of traveling from field to consumer whole and intact, conveyed a simple, uncomplicated message, that we are in the end the best judges of our own physical, mental, and emotional well-being. Living free for the conference participants translated to cutting through the rhetoric of impending doom, the blur of celebrity hype and media hysteria generated by the gluten-free industry. We sat outdoors at meals eating with gusto whole-wheat scones, turnovers, bagels, pizza, and breads washed down by wheat beers. The word *gluten* never came up. It was the most enjoyable collection of nonneurotic foodies I've ever encountered.

There was a community vibe in the air, very much in keeping with the communal character of the local grain economy. Tom Hunton, who with his wife, Sue, established Camas Country Mill in

2011 in Eugene, Oregon, talked to the assembled audience about the various ways their operation coalesced the surrounding rural folks in southern Willamette Valley in part by introducing local schoolchildren to the organic red- and white-bread wheat, spelt, emmer, rye, oats, barley, and teff that Camas was bringing back in its fields, processing in its stone gristmill, and selling locally through grocery merchants and farmer's markets. Their community-focused effort, which revived interest in the valley's history as a thriving grain area before industrialization, also brought people together to help the Huntons restore a hundred-year-old schoolhouse, he said.

His vision rekindled memories of stories I'd read about the multilayered role played by millers and bakers in villages throughout history up to the introduction of the roller mill. Darra Goldstein, professor of Russian at Williams College and founding editor of *Gastronomica*, a journal of food and culture, elaborated in her conference keynote speech. She toured us through a slide show of historical paintings; in several of them, peasants hold large loaves of bread close to their chests and slice toward themselves, not away as might be expected. "That gesture looks risky, even dangerous," she said, "but it is deliberate. It is meant to show a reverence and deep respect for bread as an intimate food that nourishes the heart and soul." Her favorite of the group—and mine—was a work by the extraordinary twentieth-century female Russian painter Zinaida Serebriakova depicting a gaunt farmer near a wheat field slicing a dark, heavy loaf the size of a large melon with eyes almost shut, as if in prayer, while beside him, eyes cast downward as well, a woman in a vivid red blouse methodically empties a jug of milk. We know he will not lose a crumb and that she will not spill a drop. We know, too, that the bread itself is a sacred bond between them.

An early Renaissance painting displayed a family gathered around a large bread oven as if in a maternity ward—and indeed, the town oven, Goldstein explained, was often used as a birthing site. "It was the only sterile, clean place in the village, so the woman going into labor crawled inside it to deliver her baby."

And from there to paintings of medieval bakeries—below-ground, in basements, so that heat would rise up to the sleeping areas. "The only light in this underworld comes from the oven, as you see. It's extremely elemental. To dismiss so much heritage by going gluten-free, well, that's giving up a lot more than gluten."

Goldstein's observations, in tandem with the artwork she chose, brought home to me the life-and-death significance of wheat and bread in society with far more impact than anything I'd read. For the first time I could feel the primal longing behind the local grain economy. It extended beyond food to a genuine human connection grounded in shared values at one of the most fractious, impersonal, fear-ridden times in our history, the current days of our lives as citizens of a chaotic world. Nothing soothes the savage soul like the smell of warm bread in the oven.

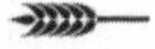

It was at the Kneading Conference West (since renamed the Grain Gathering) that I first met Washington State University's director, Stephen Jones, the plant breeder who teamed up with Dan Barber of Blue Hill restaurant at Stone Barns in New York to produce Barber's own custom variety and who is helping to reintroduce medium and small-scale organic grain farming to western Washington, which was home to 169 different wheat varieties between 1850 and 1950. There is no way to overstate Jones's importance to the artisan grain revolution in America. The Bread Lab he instituted at WSU, as one example, with its Willy Wonka array of instruments for measuring and analyzing every aspect of bread dough from starch-protein ratio and ash percentage, or mineral content, to elasticity, has now played host to Chad Robertson and hundreds of artisan bakers, breeders, and millers as well as international chefs and trainees.

"There's a whole new world of flour out there revolutionizing the way we bake," Jones said. "Freshness and variety make all the difference." He'd given me a half hour of his time toward the end of the conference, which he was also directing. By then I'd sampled that ever-changing new world in whole-grain pizzas and handmade soba noodles and wood-burning oven breads and pastries from Northwest wheat with a distinctive chocolate flavor, all served under tents set up on the sprawling grounds of the center. Sessions included making heritage wheat puff pastry, earth ovens, braided whole-wheat challah, along with tours of the Bread Lab and wheat fields—more, that is to say, than I thought I'd ever want to know about wheat and bread until I began to learn about it as an artisan craft, and then I couldn't acquire too much hands-on knowledge. I came away with my own discovery of fresh wheat's gifts: imagine eating a just-picked, perfectly ripe peach in the orchard, still sun-warmed; these baked goods consumed throughout four days put me in mind of that same unfiltered direct experience of mouthwatering, full flavor.

Nowhere does grain of any sort grow in more splendid surroundings than in Skagit Valley, where wheat stalks checkerboard with acres of multicolored tulips on the edge of the Strait of Juan de Fuca waterway just to the west, between the Olympic Mountains and snowcapped Cascades. Fields of burnished gold glint in the summer sunlight like swaths of shimmering fabric rippling beneath lush green stands of evergreen and cedar. And no one appreciates the setting more than Jones, who tells me when we meet that, like Santa Clara County—now Silicon Valley—agricultural areas to the south, closer to Seattle, got swallowed up by development as Microsoft and Amazon expanded, leaving only Skagit as the last virgin farming region in western Washington.

"Why bother to grow wheat in this area when we've got fifty million acres in the Wheat Belt and all those tons of soft white from eastern Washington being shipped to Asia?" he asks rhetorically. Then, without pause: "Because *this* was once a thriving grain area, it can be again. We're out to prove our heirloom and modern organics compete with any in flavor and performance."

Jones first met up with wheat as a breeding technician in 1977 "and just fell in love with the crop." Initially he admired it as a scientist looking only at commodity wheat. But over the years, his fondness for the grain conflicted with his uneasiness about the way it was bought and sold. Industrial giants like Cargill and General Mills typically do not own wheat acreage. Growers know the grade of their crop but not where it ends up. What they care about is yield and price. "I define commodity as, 'Did someone on a trading board in Kansas, Chicago, Minneapolis tell you what it's worth?' " says Jones. "If so, the farmer never has any idea what happens to the wheat once it leaves the farm, or gets a say in pricing. It's a commodity—with no identity." He expanded on that in an interview with *Eater*: "Whether you're a restaurant or a consumer, you should treat sourcing your grains the way you treat sourcing your meat. I look at the commodity grains like confined hogs. It's not as brutal of course, but it's a very similar system."

Jones arrived on the main campus of WSU as a wheat geneticist in 1991, working within the system, but homogenization, chemical-dependent cultivation, and poor land management continued to grate, until finally in 2008 he moved completely away from agribusiness to become director of the research center and concentrate on small, diverse, organic regional wheat farming. "We want the flavors to shine. We want the farmer to set his or her price, as they do for their tomatoes and every other crop. We also want them to know who's buying it." Growers, he explains, also want the character of heritage combined with the disease resistance and increased yields available in modern wheat, and he and his staff are advancing varieties through crossbreeding that deliver the goods in both areas.

To be successful, their varieties first have to find acceptance among end users; with that in mind, Jones joined a group of small-farm breeders who meet with chefs like Barber and bakers in New York to bring them in early in the process; breeding a new variety can span five or more years. The experiment involves gathering information on what characteristics the end users hope to find in their whole-grain flour—a flavor and performance profile—and then crossbreeding to achieve the desired customized results, with yearly tastings en route to determine if they're hitting the mark. Adjustments are made on that basis.

Targeted breeding for bakers is one of a handful of similar experiments that may or may not work out as envisioned, says Jones. He's more invested in the momentum they're gaining than in the success achieved from any one method in particular. In his long career Jones feels he spent way too much time among industry folk who view wheat as faceless, while he came to view it as the maltreated worthy stepchild of indifferent commodity traders. Around the country, he asserts, there's enough technical expertise and focused energy to reintroduce an identity to wheat that it lost more than a century ago. His dream is for states like Vermont and Maine and New York to become self-sufficient wheat-growing regions again, as in the past. Within five years or so, Jones believes, we'll see it influencing a change in the kinds of baked goods that consumers look for in places where you might not expect them to. Maybe not McDonald's, I thought to myself, but quite possibly Panera.

When I leave the conference a day later, after submerging my arms up past my elbows in a mixing bowl of dough during a bread-making class and snipping off anthers in a crossbreeding class, I pause to consider that the same species of grain, *Triticum aestivum*, responsible for the miraculous wood-fired whole-wheat pizza, boules—French rustic round loaves—and challah and such that I've enjoyed over the past few days also produces all the packaged sliced breads in supermarkets. Remarkable versatility and adaptability have always played leading roles in wheat's survival over ten thousand years—in human terms, transforming a multiple personality disorder into an asset.

And I've barely yet mentioned pasta from durum, a branch of the family with manifold identities of its own. One ingredient regularly added to the semolina produced by this wheat at the end of the nineteenth century promised to add vital nutritional properties "recommended by the most respected medical authorities for children, the sick, weak stomachs and convalescents." Its name was gluten.

13

Brainy Pasta

> Everything you see I owe to spaghetti.
>
> —Sophia Loren

The history can keep. So can the wisecracks. What you want to know is why you're not Italian—or that part of you, anyway, that is charged with the intake and digestion of durum semolina without leaving behind an inner tube of fat. Italians must cheat, you think. They're as sedentary as Americans, so it's not as if they're running up and down twenty flights of stairs at three in the morning while we're counting sheep. Somehow, despite that, they eat closer to three times as much pasta as we do and stay trim. Is it something in the water? They're one third as obese as Americans. They slip into a sleek black dress and tight-fitting pants after downing a daily bowl of pasta with no need to say "Scusi" to the scale they're stepping on.

I'll tell you why. They eat more, these Italians—sixty pounds a year for every man, woman, and child, compared to twenty-six pounds for us—but they don't eat much. Small *first* courses, a toe dip in the shallow end of the pool. And they're eating, not chomping at the bit. They sit, they take their time, they chew slowly, they swallow every bite before the next. Food is an event, not a split-second pit stop between meetings. They coat their pasta simply, with olive oil, a light blanket of tomato sauce, or a dab or two of pesto, and they shy away from bottled salad dressings, mayonnaise, prepackaged seasonings, fruit-loopy breakfast cereals, barbecue sauces, premade dinners, our entire banquet of hip-heavy favorites.

I asked Jovial Foods cofounder Carla Bartolucci, who splits her time between both countries, for her opinion. "I think people in Italy have less obesity simply because they eat seasonally, their food is less processed, and they do not normally follow trendy diets that can sway to imbalance," she told me. Bartolucci is concerned that as fast and cheap food becomes more ubiquitous, Italy's children are displaying the highest obesity level in all of Europe.

I haven't forgotten that country's gift to sudden death, tiramisu, the decadent layered mélange of whipped cream, eggs, sugar and mascarpone cheese, espresso and cocoa. If Italians were perfect in every way they wouldn't be Italian. But unlike us, they know how to walk off the occasional deliriously rich dessert.

Still, you're not entirely convinced. It can't just be a mash-up of national lifestyle and personal self-restraint. There has to be something in the soil that changes the composition of the durum wheat kernels and renders them less fattening. You've traveled through Puglia, Italy's heel, and Sicily, you've seen those endless dancing fields of durum wheat stretching out from the Tyrrhenian to the Ionian Sea and something moves you to believe there's a fundamental difference in the wheat itself, a slimming gene that dates back to Romulus and Remus. I'd be quick to buy into that myself, except that it is pure horse pucky.

Primitive Pasta

The durum grown over 1.7 million acres of North Dakota is genetically identical to durum grown in Italy, and much of it, as I'll soon explain, is what Italians eat. It's wheat that was hybridized about five thousand years ago by accident or design, a cross between emmer and a wild-grass species producing a tetraploid (*Triticum turgidum*), with twenty-eight chromosomes, not forty-two as in bread wheat (*T. aestivum*). Recent mapping of the complete wheat genome has encouraged researchers to further examine genetic material in bread wheat that may stimulate an autoimmune reaction to gluten in celiacs.

That material, on the D chromosome arm, is not present in einkorn, emmer, or durum. "Compared to hexaploid wheat, tetraploid wheat might be reduced in . . . epitopes that cause celiac disease because of the absence of the D-genome," one scientific study reports. More studies are sure to emerge. As yet there are preliminary findings; still, no definitive evidence exists to prove that semolina offers a safer choice than bread wheat for any of us who think we might be gluten-sensitive. Neither one is the staff of life: like other wheats, durum is critically low in one essential amino acid, lysine, which enables cells to metabolize energy from fats. Game meats, poultry, gelatin, eggs, milk, and ricotta cheese add the complementary amino acid.

Millers in both countries use similar techniques to separate out the endosperm that becomes semolina, and there is no difference in caloric carbohydrate content. As in bread, whole-wheat pasta contains bran and germ. It trumps refined semolina in nutritional value while getting trounced in consumer appeal, although as demand grows, manufacturers are creating firm-textured tasty products.

If durum is so high in gluten, I wondered, why doesn't its protein complex form air bubbles that capture carbon dioxide and cause bread loaves to rise. I put the question to Bradford W. Seabourn, supervisory research chemist at the USDA, who directed me to three studies focused on differences in the presence of high-molecular-weight glutenin in bread wheat compared to durum. Those glutenin subunit molecules not found in durum produce the dough's elasticity; in their absence, the gluten in semolina fails to create loaf volume.

The pasta made from durum is essentially a fuel low in sodium, low in saturated fat, with a low glycemic index in the safe zone below 55. Properly prepared—cooked firm, al dente, or "in the tooth"—semolina pasta comes in between 25 and 45, the wide range reflecting differences in shape. By comparison, a baked potato scores 85, popcorn and watermelon measure 72, and white-flour bread registers 71 on the scale.

Pasta registers a surprisingly (to me) low GI because of the physical entrapment of ungelatinized starch granules in semolina dough's sponge-like network of molecules. That apparently slows down the transport rate of carbo sugars through the gut wall.

I reached out to trusted nutritionist Julie Miller Jones for more on that, and she responded within minutes (every writer should be so fortunate). Some ungelatinized starch is not well utilized by amylase, the enzyme in flour that helps digest carbohydrates, she said. Overcooking pasta, she added, can increase the amount of gelatinized starch and raise its GI number. Miller also pointed out that the nonporous (paste-like) matrix of pasta slows absorption. "It is very different from the airy, thin cell-walled, porous structure of bread. In the latter, the amylase enzyme readily interacts with the starch and produces glucose for rapid absorption."

Francesco Pantò, director of product development at the Barilla Group in Parma, Italy, agrees. He told Christopher Wanjek of *LiveScience* that the extrusion process—in which the unleavened semolina dough is pushed through a die to give pasta tubes their shape—additionally creates "a very compact structure, which makes the carb slowly available [in the body], hence determining a slow energy release." Its strong gluten content, he added—*durum* is Latin for "hard"—prevents starch from leaching out quickly, with a greater feeling of satiation.

I came away with a reminder to myself that al dente isn't just toothy pasta, it's brainy pasta, the kind that smart people—slim Italians, for instance—eat to slow the flow of starch sugars that spike insulin levels and deposit layers of fat.

"Senza Glutine?"

By some feat of illogic I first assumed that gluten was not an issue for Italians, since they have been happily eating pasta for at least eight hundred years, and probably longer. A short time later a friend reminded me that some of the leading celiac medical experts in America studied in Italy, Stefano Guandalini and Alessio Fasano among them. When I looked into it, I learned that Italy founded its celiac association, Associazione Italiana Celiachia (AiC), thirty-five years ago, and that these physicians were trained there as specialists. I recalled Fasano telling me that he took up that specialty because it was the most popular path to pursue at his medical school. More than 150,000 Italians have been diagnosed with celiac disease. The true figure is thought to be much higher.

I'd heard and read repeatedly that American tourists who normally avoided pasta at home were discovering that they could eat it in Italy without suffering their usual bloating discomforts. (Differences in processing techniques and softer wheats are said to be primarily responsible.) But if Italians with wheat-based medical issues were new to me, they weren't to that country's food industry or national health system. As Andrew Curry reported in the *New York Times*, the Italian government gives a monthly allowance of about 100 euros ($130) to celiacs to buy specially formulated gluten-free products at the pharmacy. Curry and his gluten-intolerant wife, Jen, traveled to Genoa, Sicily, Turin, and other locales, at first concerned that they'd find nothing but salads for her to eat. Curry's sprightly article is all about the splendid array of surprising wheatless dishes that awaited, mostly corn- or chickpea flour–based, gluten-free versions of Italian standards like fusilli, not to mention gelato. "We found that Italians responded to the magic words '*senza glutine*?' not with exasperation or annoyance but with genuine concern, verging on pity."

When asked why she knew that so much of the menu was gluten-free, one server shot back, "What do you mean, how do I know? There are lots of people with food allergies. It's important to know what's in the food."

Allergies and celiac issues, *si*, but what about self-diagnosed sensitivity? I suspected Curry knew something about that as well, so I contacted him with a few questions at his home in Berlin. "I spoke with the folks at the celiac society in Italy," he responded by e-mail, "and they said gluten sensitivity is a thing there, but it makes them a little nervous. Basically, they worry that if gluten-free becomes a fad people will stop taking the medical needs of celiacs seriously. I think it's hard for Italians to imagine *voluntarily* giving up wheat, though."

He was equally articulate on the common perception that European wheat is easier to digest. "I don't know if the wheat is different, or if American food tends to be more processed. The gluten-free options here are more limited, refrigerators are smaller, and the emphasis in general is more on cooking fresh or from scratch, so there's less of the 'boxed mix' industry/market. . . . I wonder if people eating bread in Europe but not in the US are projecting a little bit, and psychosomatically assuming everything is better in Europe."

Macaroni Mythology

What better way to occupy myself for six hours on a cross-country plane ride to New York than to delve into *Pasta: The Story of a Universal Food* by Silvano Serventi and Françoise Sabban. As I plunge into the book, I can feel the stranger in the seat beside me gently listing away toward the far window. She's pegged me for the kind that might at any moment decide to share fascinating, fun pasta facts from my research on noodles and she's trapped. But no worries, I'm too engrossed. *Pasta* is so scrupulously researched that it contains over seven hundred references and eighty-odd pages alone devoted to "pasta's other homeland," China, beginning with Shi Xi's "Ode to *Bing*," an homage to Chinese wheat flatbread written in 281 CE. It occurs to me that if I really didn't like the woman seated beside me I could start with an oral recitation of this twenty-stanza poem and almost certainly impel her to leap out of the airplane long before we reached JFK.

The first myth that any pasta historian is quick to debunk involves Marco Polo's role in bringing the durum noodle back from China to Italy in 1296 after twenty-four years on the road, and introducing pasta to his fellow Venetians. Documents led researchers to believe that dried pasta made with durum found its way into Italy and then Spain four centuries earlier, when Muslims from North Africa conquered Sicily in 800 CE. Nomadic Arabs are thought to have carried it westward from Asia. Sicilians still call spaghetti "trii," derived from the Arab word for string. What Polo brought back from China was flour most likely ground from breadfruit; in his *Travels* he compared it to vermicelli and lasagna, a thin semolina crepe, which he knew all about. In America and in Italy, where all three hundred–plus forms of dried pasta (pasta *secca*), blended from ground durum, water, or eggs, are known as macaroni, there is a common misconception that the ancient Greeks and Romans were its inventors. Not so, says Clifford A. Wright in *A Mediterranean Feast*, and when it comes to pasta, feasting, anything historical and gastronomical concerning that part of the world, Wright is your man. In his book, a massive eight-hundred-page compendium of dazzling scholarship and even more remarkable recipes, he tells us that the Romans and Greeks grew and ate bread wheat, not durum.

By the fourteenth century pasta was well known throughout much of modern-day Europe. Naples in time became one of its primary manufacturing centers. Dried vermicelli and other versions made their way to Spain and France, where members of the Ashkenazic community struggled to accommodate it with Jewish law. A long discussion in the Jerusalem Talmud centers on whether boiled pasta dough should be considered unleavened bread. Needless to say, there are conflicting opinions. Pasta shows up in many cultures for a simple reason: unlike almost all other foods throughout history up to the last century, its dried version traveled without spoilage. The long shelf life has for millennia awarded dried semolina permanent residence in the larder. While pasta began as aristocratic fare, by the sixteenth century it became an inexpensive, sometimes lifesaving foodstuff for the common people, a low-cost staple in Germany and Hungary known as spaetzle, in Poland as pierogi, in Greece as orzi, among Ashkenazic Jews as kreplach dumplings, and as fideo noodles in Spain.

Founding Noodle Master

In the United States the pasta industry took root early in the nineteenth century, but it "originated with an artisanal movement that began well before the massive Italian immigration," I learned from Serventi and Sabban, the two *Pasta* authors whose journey through macaroni minutiae kept me company on the airplane. I should mention that I was heading to New York in part to hang out with a boutique pasta maker in Brooklyn; I wanted to show up at least minimally conversant on the subject. Just about the time that my eyes started to slide off the page—we were probably somewhere over the wheat fields of the Great Plains—a name popped up in the text that caused me to exclaim, out loud, "Whoa, wudda you know!"

I woke the woman beside me from a dead sleep. She lifted her eye mask, blinked a few times, and eyeballed me as if I'd just poured ice water down her back.

"Jefferson," I muttered, feeling obliged to explain. She was glancing up at the stewardess button by now. "Big pasta fan," I added. "Who knew?"

Taking the safest route to ending any conversation before it began, she nodded in silence.

"That's all for the moment," I said, more or less babbling like a street corner prophet. She waited expectantly; I wasn't the first nutcase she'd run into, but when I didn't pick up the thread she slipped her mask back in place. "Davis?" I suddenly heard her ask out of the blue. I was lost for a moment, then I put the two words together. "No," I said, "the other one, Thomas."

A brief hum-grunt in response and she was back to sleep.

Thomas Jefferson indeed. Wine buff, techno junkie, my favorite among all the founders, something of a cad, and bit of a deadbeat, but insatiably curious and thought to have imported the first pasta-making machine on American soil. While ambassador to France in the late 1780s Jefferson commissioned his secretary, William Short, to travel to Naples. Short purchased a small home version that was eventually shipped to Monticello. It was not quite what Jefferson had in mind, apparently: he wanted a large, industrial, Neapolitan pasta maker, and included his mechanical drawing and elaborate instructions on making pasta with an assist from his "maccaroni [*sic*] machine." No one knows if Jefferson's pasta maker, which was supposed to press out strands through holes in the bottom of an iron box, ever did its job. In later years Jefferson served macaroni or spaghetti that he had cut and hand-rolled into noodles from strips of dough.

Forgotten Visionary

About a century later a Kansas farm boy, Mark Alfred Carleton, grew up to be the first American who may have been entirely obsessed with wheat, according to Frederick Kaufman, the author of *Bet the Farm*. Early on he recognized that while so many varieties failed in the Great

Plains, the wheat sowed by Russian Mennonites held up against climatic, fungal, and pest devastation so relentless during the 1890s that a quarter of a million people fled Kansas. He was determined to find other varieties that performed as well or better on American soil. Carleton taught himself Russian and in 1898 set sail for Russia.

During his search on the Siberian steppe for a drought- and rust-resistant wheat that would thrive in the United States, he found Kubanka durum, a wheat one observer said could grow in hell. Finally planted by reluctant farmers in the Great Plains after strenuous campaigning by Carleton, it marked the beginning of the US durum industry and at first infuriated millers, who could not process a kernel so hard by comparison with spring varieties. The cost of retrofitting their mills dissuaded them until the following year, when black rust wiped out the spring wheat crop. Only then did they grudgingly agree to mill it, and farmers planted Kubanka as their main crop. Carleton also introduced a hard red Russian winter bread wheat, Kharkov.

By 1914, says Kaufman, half of the wheat harvested in the United States came from Carleton's varieties, more than eighty million bushels. True or not, Carleton made durum a sustainable, profitable US crop. For his troubles, the man himself never got rich or turned any kind of profit. Carleton was kicked out of government service, where he earned a meager living, on corruption charges when he borrowed money from a shady lender to pay for his daughter's infantile paralysis medical care; he lost his home and died in poverty in a foreign land, Peru. An obituary for Carleton in the November 17, 1926, edition of the *Mennonite Weekly Review* reads, "Now the strangest part of his grand and melancholy story is this: That the very qualities which made him one of the most notable of all Americans also brought him to his ultimate disaster. For he was a visionary. That was what caused him to revolutionize our western wheat industry. He was a dreamer. That was what brought him to his end."

Weathering the Elements

The dreamer died, but not the dream. Today Americans eat six billion pounds of durum pasta each year. About 80 percent comes from North Dakota, Montana, and Saskatchewan (Canada is by far the largest durum producer in North America); the remainder, "desert durum," is grown in Arizona and California, much of it processed in Italy. We ship one third of ours to Italy, Morocco, Venezuela, and a few other countries. One company alone, Barilla, buys 30 percent of its 1.4 million annual tons from American farmers.

When you give this global interchange some thought, you realize that Americans who eat pasta without any stomach or intestinal issues in Italy are probably eating durum grown in the Great Plains, as are Italians in their own country, at least as a portion of the semolina blend. In practice, semolina producers strive to present their ground durum to consumers in a warm yellow signature hue, but excessive rainy conditions leach out color, so intercontinental blending of wheats is commonplace when uncooperative weather requires adept intervention to beautify nature's bounty. Processing methods for industrial mass-market pasta do not vary between Europe and the United States.

North Dakota Wheat Commission marketing director Jim Peterson told me that although Barilla has a domestic plant in Iowa, it ships about 25 percent of domestic grain to Italy, where it gets processed and packaged and returned as finished pasta, a system employed by most international pasta companies. Isn't that enormously wasteful in fuel and energy, I asked? "It's very controversial," he replied. He clearly wasn't comfortable defending blatant carbon-footprint felons. Things were bad enough. His state's main crops, hard red spring wheat and durum, both had recently been hit hard by the climate change resulting from greenhouse-gas emissions produced in part by these manufacturers' irresponsible fuel usage. Unstable weather conditions were now spiking the price by 20 percent in the current year as supplies dwindled. "To get that deep yellow hue, high-quality durum, you need a dry July through late August, but we've been getting wet springs followed by humid summers, plus fungal diseases like fusarium and verticillium that have hammered yield."

Just about everyone wants their semolina processed at North Dakota Mill and Elevator in Grand Forks, the nation's most prestigious durum processor and the only grain mill in the country owned by the people of the state, not privately held. Back in 1919 a socialist organizer, A. C. Townley, formed the National Non-Partisan League and rallied North Dakota's exploited rural folk to take ownership of their farmland—rich in loam but not in profits for farmers. Gaining wealth from their labors, freight tycoons and Minneapolis investors and financiers had prospered by owning all of the rail lines and elevators and mills. Within a few years Townley's political recruits won every statewide office and controlled the legislature. His coalition soon dissolved, but not before making the state's largest grain mill a public entity; its profits now feed North Dakota's general fund, and its operation requires no taxpayer money. Liberal bloviators routinely highlight the irony of a state-owned enterprise thriving in a heavily conservative state that has voted Republican in twenty-five of thirty-one presidential elections.

I skipped that topic in my conversation with Peterson and asked instead if the locavore movement had penetrated North Dakota's wheat industry. "There's a definite trend," he told me. "As more of their food gets processed, people want to know more and more where it comes from." He included himself and his wife. I knew from talking with artisanal pasta makers around the country that North Dakota Mill regularly supplied much of the durum they used.

That holds true for Sfoglini, one of the first boutique manufacturers I plan to visit in New York, where revived state local grains now include bread wheat, against long odds, but no durum. The New York summers are much too humid. According to *Serious Eats*, an informative, popular online foodie magazine as well as numerous social media sites, the New York locavore grain movement is "exploding" in popularity. I'm eager to learn more. Living in California, I find it all too tempting to convince myself that anything and everything purely healthful, morally righteous, super-conscientious, spiritually advanced, and ultra-natural transpires within our Golden State's borders.

Not quite. The thriving local heritage revival—local, by the way, also includes regional—in New York and New England as elsewhere, belies that parochial view. The Kneading Conference West, in fact, began in Skowhegan, Maine, in 2007 under the leadership on Maine Grain Alliance director Amber Lambke, before branching out to create the Skagit Valley West Coast version.

Whole vs. White

How do nutritional differences between whole-wheat durum flour and semolina (ground endosperm) stack up against whole-wheat and refined white-bread flour, I wondered. To learn more, I browse the

Oldways website (oldwayspt.org). On it Cynthia Harriman, director of Food and Nutrition, lays out in detail the case for pasta as a staple of the Mediterranean Diet that contributes to reducing both coronary artery disease and issues bundled together as the metabolic syndrome, a combination of high blood pressure, high cholesterol, and obesity. Harriman, whom I've spoken with at length, has put together a comprehensive, updated archive of nutritional and general information on all grains at wholegrainscouncil.org, in a clear and concise format. (It's all favorable; the site is funded by the wheat industry but more factual than promotional.)

The basic durum versus bread flour question I searched on, however, comes up empty. I find an answer I wasn't looking for on Rodale's Prevention website. In a "Health Food Face-Off," Prevention puts whole-wheat durum up against gluten-free spaghetti. It wins, but narrowly—in five out of nine categories. Most of the differences are marginal, fat and carb content and such. But gluten-free contains twice the calcium and iron—no mention of whether it's been added back, a likely scenario—and whole wheat contains close to four times the fiber and twice the protein. Livestrong, the nonprofit organization that supports people in managing and surviving cancer, reports about twice as much fiber in whole wheat as enriched pasta, as well as more magnesium and phosphorus. As in bread, levels of fiber, the meal of choice for friendly gut microbes, account for the most important difference. As a better health choice whole wheat wins.

14 New York Noodles

Life is a combination of magic and pasta.
—Federico Fellini

What to make of all this? It comes down yet again not so much to what is good for you but what is good for you that you will actually look forward to eating. That I take to be the singular advantage of locally grown and milled organic whole-wheat pasta. Stephen Colbert might even ask for seconds. I've sampled Community Grains' rendition and a few others, and I'm eager to explore more versions. Too eager, perhaps. At the moment, on this early morning in January 2014, I'm up to my exposed frozen ankles in slushy snow as I try to make my way from a Metro subway station on Flatbush Avenue in Brooklyn to the Sfoglini pasta company, half a mile away, feeling the penetrating chill of one of New York's worst blizzards in a winter from hell. I can't see beyond three feet at best; the rest of the world dissolves into a white swirling blur. Gusts from the East River blow sheets of horizontal snow into my face and my ears and down my neck.

As the wind howls and moist snowflakes splat and stick on my eyelids, I flash back to my childhood growing up in New England. We used to pray for this kind of miserable wet snow as kids because the snowballs you could make from it became instant missiles of destruction, hard-packed and heavy and capable of exploding with kinetic force against the front window of a passing car, causing the driver to swerve or screech to a skidding stop as we dove behind a hedge.

I was the snowball thrower; now I'm the windshield. My mother told me as a boy to wear my galoshes but she didn't tell me to move to California and walk around in slip-on loafers that don't quite do the job on this trek up snow-blitzed Flatbush Avenue. By the time I reach the former Pfizer building where Sfoglini is located, half an hour later, I'm permafrosted. What I'd give for a hot, steaming cup of coffee, and good luck finding it anywhere near here. But wait. That roasty aroma—I know it at once, we all do, it's in our DNA. At first I suspect I'm hallucinating. As I shake off snow and I dry my eyes, however, I find that I'm stationed before a wall of logo tiles, the building's index. Surrounding the Sfoglini Pasta Shop logo with room number are People's Pops, makers of local fruit ice pops; also McClure's small-batch pickles, Madécasse chocolates, Liddabit Sweets, Kombucha Brooklyn, a roster of boutique food and beverage makers including . . . fresh-drip organic coffee. I've stumbled onto eight floors of culinary artisanal start-ups in a building where Pfizer once centrifuged compounds that dissolved kidney stones.

I soon locate the fresh-coffee vendor, warm my hands and throat, and let the hot liquid slide down, a miracle cure, as I make my soggy way up to Sfoglini.

Co-owner Steve Gonzalez is busy when I enter, working dough from a feeder through a bronze disc about six inches across with repetitive curlicue patterns inscribed into it. Extruded accordion-shaped tubes emerge and spill into a basin. The die resembles an Indian mandala. Much of Sfoglini's single room has been given over to storage, refrigeration, and drying. The pasta machinery itself occupies little space. I'm aware of wind-blown snow rattling the windows, but to Gonzalez it's simply background music. When he takes a break, we talk. "The name? Ladies in Bologna who make pasta by hand are called *sfoglini*," he explains. Freshly extruded pasta spreads out near us on racks in a heated area where they will air-dry for forty-eight to ninety-six hour.

As an expression of the owners' commitment to bringing forward a noble tradition, the company's Italian name seems a reasonable choice, but better still if you can pronounce it. The *g* is silent and the *o* is long, so Sfoglini rhymes with "low beanie." A former chef and pasta maker, Gonzalez, in his early thirties, learned his trade at a three-star Michelin restaurant in Spain and as a chef in Italy before teaming up with former creative director and graphic designer Scott Ketchum about two years ago.

The partners—Scott handles brand development and operations—envisioned opening a restaurant with a side pasta business, but when funding proved difficult they decided to focus on fresh wholesale pasta, and when that proved less successful as a retail item than their dried version, they shifted their product line to whole-wheat blends and short runs of seasonal dried, flavored varieties. Fresh ingredients pulverized in a Vitamix blender include nettles, beets, chili peppers, and an "everything bagel" pasta that combines bagel bits with sesame seeds, garlic, and onion—sufficiently quirky and tasty to create a New York buzz and gain media attention. (Sfoglini continues to sell fresh pasta to restaurants.)

It helps that Scott's wife works at a brewery, which inspired them to seek out spent grain from beer brewing; ever adventurous, they later added a flavored pasta derived from Red Hook Winery grape skins before the winery got whacked by Hurricane Sandy, as well as tomato leaves and other local farm ingredients like late-season basil. Sfoglini's nonseasonal specialty pastas blend New York whole heritage wheat from Don Lewis's Wild Hive Farm and Mill in Hudson Valley and North Dakota durum (a 60:40 ratio) in imaginative origami shapes such as radiator, reginetti, zucca, and spaccatelle, each requiring its own Italian bronze die.

"Are you using Wild Hive's flour to support local grain?" I asked.

"No, I'm more about taste than I am about anything. It's got amazing flavor. We like to keep it local but the product comes first. We're also now experimenting with stone-ground desert durum from Hayden Flour Mill in Arizona."

When you dry pasta slowly, staying at or under 105 degrees Fahrenheit, Gonzalez continues, you preserve flavors and nutrition. "Over one hundred five degrees you start to denature the vitamins, which is why they add back riboflavin and niacin to semolina in commercial supermarket pastas. They dry with high heat for economy reasons, but you pay a big price as a consumer."

Slow air-drying by contrast adds to labor costs; it's one of several reasons local-grain pastas cost two or three times as much, Gonzalez explains. Added to that at the moment is the rising price of durum. "Even in North Dakota our grain cost has risen 20 percent over the past six months."

I think back to my conversation with Jim Peterson and the ricochet effect of drought conditions brought about by climate change, changes that make North Dakota's farmlands now more amenable than ever to GMO soy and corn than durum and hard red.

"We're tying to hold our price level, and we changed to a low flat shipping rate for customers on our website," Gonzalez tells me, "but we're feeling it."

In truth I give little thought to my experience at Sfoglini when I return home, after depositing a few boxes of its whole-wheat blended spiral radiators and fusilli in our pantry. One early evening a few weeks later, when I'm walking into the kitchen, I find Bonnie stirring olive oil with a scoop of parsley into an al dente saucepan of organic filigree Sfoglini pasta. "It looked interesting," she remarks. A short time later we add a light sprinkling of pecorino, then look at each other as we swallow our first taste, and eat a second forkful without a passing a word between us. We have the same palate. "It is as good as I think it is, isn't it?" she says at length.

I nod.

It is. Subtle yet intense, silken yet toothy. A hint of gravel and sweet savory accents arrive in the same bite, a delightful complication of flavors. The texture is springy, alive. My taste buds catch on before my overeducated left brain catches up, and I find myself consuming half a bowl before I pause.

Extruding Value

Pasta Sonoma does not need the business. Or the headaches. Extruding whole-wheat durum requires special dies, longer drying time, and processing that slows down production lines. Don Luber and his wife and business partner, Susan, have been private-labeling a wide range of semolina pasta products for a large innovative national grocery chain for more than two decades. Their company trucks in semolina from Montana milled by General Mills to its compact factory located about forty miles north of San Francisco in a small industrial complex in Rohnert Park, south of Santa Rosa. Specialty natural-flavored varieties like lemon-pepper fettuccine and sweet potato fusilli have become signature products, and Luber has customized Pasta Sonoma's equipment to turn out ten thousand pounds of finished product a day. A laminating machine creates thin sheets sliced into ribbons of various widths that are dried in a row of large, custom-made wooden enclosures, each individually controlled and modified to his specifications.

But a short time back, about two years ago, Bob Klein from Community Grains and Joe Vanderliet and Monica Spiller, the doyenne of California heritage grains, came knocking on Pasta Sonoma's door. Spiller, Luber soon learned, pioneered the planting of heritage California wheats from the USDA seed bank by organic farmers and founded the Whole Grain Connection to sell and give away the Ethiopian Blue Tinge and other grains they harvested. With her late husband, Eugene Spiller, a physician, Monica wrote a book on the health benefits of fiber; as a former analytical chemist, she laid out the scientific reasoning behind whole wheat's nutritious advantages to Luber. He was duly impressed. The three were at Pasta Sonoma to explore his interest in helping to fabricate products from small lots of organic varieties like Sonora and Espresso, once popular in California before dwarf wheat overran the state. Staffed and equipped to process thousands of pounds daily for national retailers, yet small by industry standards, and, most of all, potentially accessible to artisan entrepreneurs, Pasta Sonoma occupies a unique position in the industry.

Luber tells me that the convictions of those dedicated visitors "made me a believer in the value of local whole wheat and I wanted to hitch our wagon to something we believed in." Klein said he had lined up Whole Foods for his Community Grains products, and that, Luber says, got his attention. I am visiting the plant after thawing out and returning from New York, sitting across from him and general manager Cindy Riddle in the company's conference room. Trim and tanned and remarkably spry at seventy-five, Luber spins tales with animated zeal in the forceful, booming baritone of an announcer breaking news stories at eleven. He knew that Pasta Sonoma would have to invest in equipment, including costly bronze extrusion dies, he tells me, also that local grain production would initially represent only about 5 percent at most of his total business. What he didn't know, he adds, is how different and difficult processing that wheat into pasta would be. "A *huge* difference!" Luber discovered the absorption rate and amount of water required for whole-wheat durum dough to be nothing like the demands for semolina.

"A pain in the ass, basically, is what you're saying."

"Exactly!"

"So why take it on?"

"Here's why. It was the entire wheat as God made it. You're not taking out the germ or the bran, all the micronutrients are in it, stone ground, it makes complete sense. That's how I got introduced to whole grain. Also it gave us an opportunity to come out and talk about ourselves as innovators producing new varieties of flour from heirloom wheats."

That, of course, is not an option as a private-label manufacturer.

I'd been alerted in advance by Bob Klein that Luber tended to be protective and withholding about his business dealings and production methods, but when I called and talked with Riddle about my interest in checking out an established commercial pasta manufacturer willing to stretch out for artisanal clients, she became an ally and gave her boss some background on me; he readily agreed to an interview. The guy I'm sitting across from at the moment, and will spend half a day with, is anything but guarded. Confident and amiable, Luber airs out his views without hesitation. For a decade or more Luber and his wife promoted their own Pasta Sonoma brand at fifteen or more trade shows a year. The wealth of hard-won industry knowledge Luber acquired he was only too willing to pass on to Klein, who decided instead to strike out on his own. "Community Grains is still working to gain a foothold three years in, but I believe in what they're all about. Sometimes," Luber remarks with a shrug, "you have to do things yourself."

As a father whispering the wisdom of my experience into the deaf ears of our children during their teenage years, I get it.

While Luber's appraisal may prove correct, I wouldn't bet against Klein finding a way to turn a profit in the large, expanding specialty-foods market. He's a guy who, with his wife, Maggie, opened the small restaurant, Oliveto, thirty years ago in Oakland that hung on through tough times to become a Bay Area food lovers' mecca. He's used it as a test kitchen for grains from heritage polenta to wheat and beyond that no one else was willing to explore, or even cared about—and the dishes that have emerged, I can attest, are phenomenally rich, uniquely flavorful, and satisfying. As with so many other enterprises, marketing and funding will play a decisive role in determining Community Grains' fate. The pasta that Luber produces for him, meanwhile, speaks eloquently for itself.

Friend or Foe?

Delving into semolina and durum, I'm reminded yet again that wheat in America seems destined to lead a double life. Amy's

Kitchen, a Petaluma-based purveyor of organic foods, has been growing at 23 percent a year, and the company now worries that its organic wheat sources aren't adequate to meet increasing demand for its noodle products. Since word got out about the artisan bent of Pasta Sonoma, scores of small growers have contacted the company to make whole-wheat pasta from their durum. "I've been astonished at the number," Luber says. "We had no idea of the scope."

At the same time gluten-free products continue to sell in record number, even though in many, if not most, cases, they deposit higher levels of refined sugars in our bloodstreams than their whole-wheat counterparts and offer minimal nutritive value at considerably more expense. Wheat flour consumption has fallen to a twenty-two-year low, and anti-gluten's most influential proponents who proclaim that wheat "is silently destroying your brain" (David Perlmutter) and that it is "the world's most destructive dietary ingredient" (William Davis) continue to influence the eating habits of thousands of converts.

Summing Things Up

After more than a year of investigating the grain from a variety of perspectives, in the process becoming intimately involved with it as an avid home baker, what I've discovered is that wheat isn't getting a fair shake. It is being maltreated as a commoditized product by an industry that mills less than 5 percent of it whole and makes no effort to foster varieties of the grain that emphasize flavor, texture, those nuances and discoveries we look for in foods that we enjoy. Its legion of medical adversaries do us a great favor if they scare any of us off another helping of refined white flour in any form, from doughnut to bagel, no argument there. But they attack all wheat with an approach they would never apply to their medical practice, not if they wanted it to stay in business. Imagine for a moment that as a new patient you sat down and the first words out of the doctor's mouth were, "Stop what you're doing, stop right now! You're killing yourself!"

Before he or she knew anything about you. Before that physician began an exam or even learned your name. Because it didn't matter, he or she had an agenda and it applied to one and all. That catch-all approach describes wheat's most vociferous and most influential adversaries. Should we consider each a quack, then? No, but not a medical professional interested in reading the fine print, either—your test results, for instance. A pulpit belongs in a church or synagogue, not a medical office.

That's what I came to make of the anti-gluten, anti-carb faction after reading and seeing these alarmists in action. They approach wheat with a blanket indictment, with no interest in or patience for different processing and cultivation methods that make all the difference. It follows that they entirely ignore any research or techniques that might weaken their arguments.

Chief among them is the sourdough process, as I was to learn. If you're on the gluten-sensitive bandwagon and you have resigned yourself to never eat wheat again, whole or refined, bread or pasta or pastry, you may be in for a pleasant surprise. Some wheats are less risky than others, and some are not risky at all—extremely beneficial, in fact—regardless of the hyperbole based on largely unsubstantiated cautionary warnings. If you miss the crunch and the chewiness and the nutlike aroma that only true wheat delivers, you owe it to yourself to explore the microbial wonders and delicious mysteries of sourdough.

15

Sins of Omission

> Let things taste the way they are.
>
> —Alice Waters

You can't write about the perils of eating bread wheat and ingesting its gluten and carbohydrates without bringing fermentation into the conversation, for the same reason that you can't write about automobiles without considering the engine. Fermentation powers wheat; water is the fuel source and flour is the medium. There isn't a single reference to long or short fermentation, sprouting, soaking, or sourdough in the index of *Wheat Belly* or *Grain Brain*. Whether or not these sins of omission are deliberate, they mount up to an overall rejection of any approach that threatens to challenge the author's verdict.

For reasons of their own, wheat-bashers like William Davis and David Perlmutter do not consider the role or effect of dough-making speed, or how quickly or deliberately fungal and bacterial microorganisms metabolize the starch sugars in flour and convert them to gases, alcohol, and acids. But that rate of conversion, and the kind of yeasts used to facilitate it, directly affect how well you digest the end product and how well that dough treats you in return. They also determine whether you receive the bread's full nutritional benefits and if your gut pumps glucose into your bloodstream with the force of a firehouse or metes it out at a safe rate.

What about the teeming beneficial bacteria in your gut, those hundred trillion microbes that make up your microbiome? You can't leave them out of the conversation, either. The gut's bacteria total two to three pounds of your body weight. Long fermentation as well as sprouting and soaking allow the microflora adequate time to perform their natural functions. These processes are so common in nature that even squirrels bury their nuts to ferment them. By contrast, commercial yeasts fast-pedal the bread's absorption rate. Consumers pay the tab, says Panera Bread's head baker, Tom Gumpel, the man responsible for overseeing the daily output of close to two thousand bakery-cafés. "It does an incredible disservice to the quality of bread, in my eyes. Manufactured yeast, not machines alone, screwed this whole thing up. Instant-acting yeast puts off alcoholic fermentation versus the acidic fermentation you get from sourdough." Nothing good comes from it: "You lose taste, flavor and the bioavailability of nutrients, just for openers."

Time matters, according to Gumpel. "We're not cows. We don't have four stomachs, one just to break down grass. What makes grains some of the healthiest food on earth is the value that comes from sprouting and fermenting them at length; *their* length, not ours."

There are foods you eat, such as sprouted wheat, he continues, that, when you eat them you actually see a change in your body. Along with sourdough, sprouting—germinating wheat berries for two or three days in advance of baking—ranks as one of Gumpel's favorite "pre-consumption" methods; he now uses sprouted wheat along with spelt, rye, and oats for Panera's grain bagel flats. On his blog, *Wheat Belly*'s Davis responds with characteristic disdain to a woman's question about sprouting's merits: "It is folly to believe that such a process as simply allowing the seed to germinate somehow disables all the bad potential of modern wheat."

Folly? Maybe not. The germination process activates enzymes that are proven to break down gluten proteins and carbohydrates. Sprouting also releases phytase and amylase. Phytase unlocks phosphorous and other minerals bound up by phytic acid. Amylase makes the plant material more readily digestible by humans. Research studies indicate that enzymatic germination effectively detoxifies gluten molecules. "Germinating wheat enzymes reduce the toxicity of wheat gliadin," a 2009 study in *Annals of Medicine* reported. Biopsies on the subjects' small intestinal mucosa confirmed the findings.

Gumpel is one among an army of artisan bakers, nutritionists, and other health professionals who argue that quick-acting yeast allows no time for microbial warriors to do their job, a significant part of which is to disarm gluten molecules while preserving their elasticity and extensibility. Mass production compresses a full-length movie into a three-minute trailer. Just as no one has yet invented a better seed than nature, no one has succeeded in condensing the time span for the natural fermentation of wheat's native yeasts and bacteria without zapping our blood sugar levels and doing collateral damage. We're adaptive. Our bodies adjust and carry on, but that toxic stress accumulates. Why not choose a healthier alternative? It's a question being asked more frequently as the benefits of Old World artisan techniques gain increased media attention.

Common Grain Sense

For thousands of years many cultures around the planet have employed sprouting and other "pre-digestive" techniques to neutralized grains' enzyme inhibitors, lectins (nature's pesticides that bind carbohydrates), and anti-nutrients; predigested foods range from Japanese *mochi* (long-soaked rice) to Russian *tolokno* (soaked oats) to Indian dal to soaked cracked wheat, bulgur, in the Mideast. All involve moistening grains externally to jump-start the alimentary canal's enzymatic activity. Pre-chewing from parent to offspring has always been common among apes and in many animal species, also among humans in some cultures, to transfer saliva enzymes that break down starches and improve infant digestion. An ancient Egyptian medical papyrus instructs mothers to pre-masticate food as a remedy for children.

Soaking in an acidic environment such as yogurt or buttermilk for twenty-four hours neutralizes phytic acid. When wheat berries sprout in water for two or three days, enzymes and chemicals break down large protein chains; germination also makes vitamins A, B, and C more accessible as it releases iron, potassium, and calcium. Alvarado Street Bakery and Ezekiel Bread make sprouted wheat and multigrain breads that contain no flour. The full flavors of grain, for anyone new to them, can be a revelation.

The folk kitchen wisdom behind these techniques may be short on chemistry but long on common sense, a phrase that after all takes its name from a sensible approach to common activities like eating. That proceeds from trial and error, from closely observed cause and effect. In diverse cultures common grain sense teaches that a long ferment, usually from twelve to twenty-four hours and often performed in an organized series of steps, hastens comfortable digestion.

Numerous scientific research papers confirm these benefits and restate them in microbiological terms. Published in 2007 in the peer-reviewed *Applied and Environmental Microbiology*, one study found that long fermentation in wheat bread reduced gluten levels from 75,000 parts per million (ppm) to 12, way below the 20 ppm that is considered gluten-free. In a 2010 Italian clinical study on sourdough's effect on gluten levels published in *Clinical Gastroenterology and Hepatology*, patients with a diagnosis of celiac disease who took part were separated into two groups: one group received partially hydrolyzed wheat flour while the patients in the second group, unlike the other, received baked goods completely degraded by the lactic acid bacteria (LAB) found in sourdough. Those patients had no clinical complaints, and their celiac-related antibodies did not increase. The researchers concluded that "a sixty-day diet of baked goods made from hydrolyzed wheat flour, manufactured with sourdough lactobacilli and fungal proteases, was not toxic to patients with CD."

Biopsies for the second group revealed a change in their intestinal lining, although those patients had no clinical complaints. But the most significant change showed up in the third group. Blood levels for immune markers that signal an adverse reaction to wheat did not rise for the celiac patients who ate baked goods made from wheat flour fully broken down by sourdough's lactic bacteria; after sixty days, biopsies on each participant showed no intestinal lining deterioration.

What to make of that? "Food processing by selected sourdough lactobacilli and fungal proteases [enzymes that help to break down proteins] may be considered an efficient approach to eliminate gluten toxicity," the Italian researchers modestly conclude. While these results add to the argument that the age-old way of long-fermenting bread reduces the toxicity of gluten molecules, a word to the wise: in no way are the researchers implying that a grocery store or artisanal bakery loaf of sourdough—or wheat in any form—is safe to eat for anyone diagnosed as a celiac sufferer. They prepared the bread used for this study with specially selected, potent fungal proteases unavailable to us as consumers, and only a small number of patients participated. To make any credible broad generalizations, a larger test group of subjects will be required. What to take away, in my view, is cautious optimism.

The study's restrained, sober tone comes across as refreshing tonic relief from the scaremonger harangues of the anti-gluten faction. When I reached one of its authors, Marco Gobbetti, a distinguished professor of microbiology at the University of Bari in Italy who has published over 150 papers on related topics, he told me that the 2010 research project and another his team recently completed demonstrate without any doubt that "long fermentation makes the bread more digestible." He's working with an Italian bakery hoping to market a gluten-safe wheat bread. "But how will it rise if there's so little gluten in it?" I asked. "That we don't yet know," he replied with a sigh. We both laughed.

Under the microscope gluten amino acid molecules resemble tangled, knotted fishing lines. In sourdough, given sufficient time, amylase enzymes break down the starch as the lactic bacteria untangle and degrade these long polymer chains. The degradation process offers hope to some who consider themselves gluten sensitive and long for the firm tooth-tug and jaw-churn of real bread with a soulful yearning that no mealy soft rice flour, tapioca starch, guar, and xanthan gum surrogate can begin to mollify.

My wife, for one, used to dip slices of sponge-webbed, crusty-coated fresh sourdoughs into pools of extra-virgin olive oil with a look of pure bliss. She for many months continued to bypass that sublime experience with the resolve of a religious convert. It was Bonnie's gluten neck, as you'll recall, that launched my foray into the world of wheat while she took an alternate path and avoided glutenized grains in all forms. She thought she'd adjusted to her withdrawal and so did I. But neither of us factored in the beckoning power of baking bread.

Scaling Down

Pity the man who can't read his own bathroom scale. Or can, but won't believe what it's telling him. I'd been keeping close tabs for years on the amount of store-bought bread I ate; as I grew older, I noticed that it stuck to me with increasing frequency. Now, a few months into my book research, I was making and eating about a loaf of my own whole-wheat sourdough a week, more bread than I would normally consume in eight weeks or more. Homemade sourdough's lactic and acetic acids, the ones that came along to put spunk and bounce into the bread on our table, keep the bread fresh for up to ten or twelve days and make it a dangerous temptation each time you walk past the cutting board in the kitchen. My public rationale for becoming an ardent bread maker revolved around the notion that to understand the many moods of wheat, I had to dance with it arm in arm and study its moves at close range. Bonnie was not for a moment fooled. No one has ever had to remind her that she married an obsessive.

In my days as a Pinot Noir winemaker, after twenty straight

hours in the winery I'd crawl into bed at 4:00 a.m. during crush with shriveled grape clusters lodged in my ears. I napped in the vineyard between prunings. Although I'd traveled from grapes to grain, I still carried that gene. Bonnie knew my total-immersion inclinations only too well. What puzzled her, though, was a change in my physical being.

"Have you been skipping lunch while you write during the day?" she asked as we sat down for dinner one night.

"Nope."

"Are you sure? When we came back from Venice you were carrying all that black ink cuttlefish pasta around your waist like extra baggage. Where did it go?" I heard something rare and distinctive in her tone: a trace of envy.

I paused and thought about it. "I have no idea," I said, "but now that you bring it up, my pants do fit a little loose lately."

"And you feel okay?"

"Great!"

"So I shouldn't worry?"

Maybe it was the way she started scanning me with her jade green don't-miss-much eyes, as if I were hiding an important secret too valuable to share—something touched a nerve. Or maybe it was the mirror sending back images of a man suspiciously shedding love handles. I can't say, but I was motivated to dig our digital bathroom scale out from the cabinet under the sink. I'd paid so little attention to my weight for so long that I found I had to replace the scale's dead batteries. My wife, too, never used it. I should explain that I've been running for years, not fast and not far, about three miles four times a week, with increasing gratitude as running partners over the decades have blown out their knees. That, in company with upper body exercises, has kept me fit. Fit is really all I cared about; weight didn't matter.

But as I started to keep a log once a week, not at all convinced I was getting a correct reading, I discovered that if the numbers didn't lie, I was slowly and steadily continuing to eat sourdough and drop pounds. "I think you should write *The Grain Frame Diet*," Bonnie suggested at one point. Was there a slight edge in her tone? What wasn't I telling her? I did indeed seem to be developing a reverse wheat belly. Somewhere along the way I came upon a study cited by Dr. Joseph Mercola: "When rats were given lactic acid bacteria from birth through adulthood," he writes, "they put on significantly less weight than other rats eating the same high-calorie diet. They also had lower levels of minor inflammation, which has been associated with obesity." I'm still digesting news of my gut kinship with skinny rodents.

Free at Last

After many months on her wheat-free regimen, one early June day Bonnie made a request at breakfast: Would I mind toasting her a slice of my homemade bread as well? She asked that in a casual tone that revealed just a glimpse of yearning tucked beneath it. The nutty fragrance of a dawn bake filled the air. Something in her voice told me to stay cool, although a crash of cymbals sounded in my inner ear as she chewed and swallowed her first mouthful of wheat in half a year, my newest sourdough loaf.

How to describe her reaction? You know the moment—it's when the iron gate of the penitentiary slams shut behind the newly released prisoner. She lifts her head, closes her eyes, and breathes in free air once again with a smile so radiant, it outshines the sun above.

"This," Bonnie exclaimed, "is *bread.*" From the glint in her eye and the lusty joy in that exclamation, I wouldn't have been surprised if she picked up the loaf in both hands and ate the entire thing in one sitting. In the days that followed, my bread seemed to thaw her out from a long winter of the soul. Her mood brightened. Once she realized she was experiencing no negative reactions—a returning gluten neck, for instance, or fatigue, joint pains, constipation, thickening hips, mental fog, skins rashes, or carbo-induced sugar spikes and crashes—she began eating one or two slices every day, gleefully.

About eight weeks later she asked, "Do you notice anything different about me?" This is always a treacherous question for a husband. There's one correct answer and most often you know it too late, only after she tells you. But this time Bonnie helped by spinning around slowly, hands on hips.

"Your waist," I said with total assurance. It was a wild stab based on immediate clues, but you don't ever want to respond in that situation with a question of your own, as in, "Can you give me a hint?"

She nodded. "I've dropped the last five pounds." That was followed by a triumphant smile. To me and the world at large she was never overweight to begin with. It was a fool's errand, I knew, to point that out.

These final five turn out to be not just any five. They are the ones epoxied to your skeletal structure that follow you into the afterlife.

"Very impressive! Are you working with a new gym trainer?"

"No. I've stopped grazing," Bonnie said. "It didn't happen while

I was non-gluten. I still snacked. But your sourdough fills me up without weighing me down. I just eat at meals now."

That got me to thinking. I've always been a grazer, too. Not so much, though, since baking my own sourdoughs. In fact, hardly at all. I suspect that the presence of whole fiber and lactic acid bacteria play a role in that. The breads are organic whole wheats with spelt, einkorn, and organic dark rye and white in supporting roles, customized versions of classic formulas from Andrew Whitley, Chad Robertson, King Arthur Flour baking director Jeffrey Hamelman, Peter Reinhart, and others. (My very own Final Five Sourdough recipe I include in Appendix A.)

Over the months that followed, Bonnie checked out a limited number of whole-wheat foods like Community Grains and Sfoglini pasta and added them into her diet without fanfare or digestive problems. As I write, there are two homemade loaves crackling in our double ovens. Bonnie's ex-husband, Jacques, pops in more frequently these days, I've noticed. He's glad to see me but gladder to see my bread. "Like what I grew up on," he says after a third slice. It's a bald lie—he grew up in flatbread Morocco, but every guy finds his own way to compliment the chef.

Alive and Welcome

I don't mistake anecdotal evidence for trustworthy data, but what you can take away from my experience is that at a personal level I discovered a new and immensely rewarding relationship with wheat. It wasn't an infatuation of the adolescent-tingle variety, the hopeless, stuttering, stammering paralysis that grips you when your beloved suddenly appears and so much blood rushes to your head, or away from it, that you become tipsy and breathless before your eyes can focus. No, this was the intoxicating swoon of a more languorous, nineteenth-century romance novel. With deep affection I watched my sourdough starters bubble up and my doughs transform from soupy slush to tight, springy globes. The hazelnut scent of baking dough brought a warm smile, also a sense of contentment, and the radiant sheen of a foxy reddish-brown crust fresh from the oven filled me with joy, as did the sight of its scored top quadrants rising up like miniature windswept curling waves.

The rewards of making sourdough at home, I learned, are all the more satisfying for being well-earned. You don't, as mentioned, toss a few ingredients into a bread machine and saunter off. As I explained when I chronicled my earlier *I Love Lucy* debacle, touch is everything. With practice your hands in the mixing bowl send back messages on your progress that guide you from start to finish.

By contrast, packaged commercial sourdough breads—not local artisan loaves—arrive at their tanginess through shortcut methods. Various acids—acetic, malic, and fumaric—are added to traditionally yeasted breads; longer fermentation, with all of its health benefits, is not part of the equation.

In principle, the sourdough starter you add as the dough's leavening ignition switch is as basic as flour plus water plus air plus time plus luck. Recipes include potato broth, pineapple juice, grape skins, apple skins, milk, yogurt, and probably a jellied spider or two if you looked hard enough. Some of them attempt to give you increased access to wild yeast, others to a bounty of bacterial allies, when filtered water and unrefined flour—rye is the best—do it all. Every microbe you need is in the air you breathe or the flour you convert.

Sourdough microflora originate in the soil. Flying insects, as a best guess, inoculate the crop since that flora grows on the grain stalks. Every region delivers its own variation of yeast and bacteria. Common bakers' terms signify the essential nature of an active healthy starter culture: you do not simply mix in water and flour every day as it develops, you *feed* it. You don't simply dump in more after it gets going. You *refresh* it. It's alive.

When, after a few failed attempts, you come down one morning to find your lumpy wet dough bubbling away like the La Brea Tar Pits, as I did, you may indulge in strutting your own cleverness, but in your heart you recognize that it is just as likely fairies, pixies, and sprites visited by night to wave their wands and transform that stagnant puddle of goop into a pulsating porridge.

What you have done is to create a unique medium for the symbiotic interaction between a specialized yeast fungus, *Candida milleri*, and a dominant species of lactic bacteria, *Lactobacillus sanfranciscensis*. Normally yeasts and bacteria compete for the same sugars. But in sourdough—and as far as I know, only sourdough—they form a friendly alliance. The *C. milleri* yeast in the flour does not metabolize maltose, which the lactobacilli gobble up, while enzymes and *L. sanfranciscensis* release glucose and fructose sugars in the starch that are metabolized by this and the other strains of yeast that are present.

By excreting glucose, the *Lactobacillus sanfranciscensis* lactobacilli conserve the maltose for themselves as they produce alcohol and lactic and acetic acid, the souring agent. For full flavor, both need to be present. Sourdough's *Candida milleri* yeast survives in a low acidic pH environment (most yeasts do not) and it converts the sugars it digests into carbon dioxide and ethanol. That escaping CO_2

gas, trapped by elastic gluten, forms the bread's air pockets. These conversions require time, plenty of it, at a suitable temperature range.

The net result, in plain English, is a bread that delivers sensational taste and texture rewards. It is also a bread that for non-celiac gluten-sensitive individuals may be easily digestible. There is no certainty in any of this, but there seems to be a reasonable possibility. I suggest asking your local artisan bakers for their thoughts on how their customers respond to long fermentation.

The Sourdough Solution

> Are we really all going to spend our last years avoiding bread, especially now that bread in America is so unbelievably delicious?
>
> —Nora Ephron

About forty-five years ago, working at a USDA laboratory in Albany, California, two microbiologists, Frank Sugihara and Leo Kline, discovered and named the *Lactobacillus sanfranciscensis* bacteria and identified the significant other yeast strain in that model relationship. Sugihara and Kline found that the lactobacilli outnumber yeasts in sourdough by 100 to 1, also that *Candida milleri* yeast and lactic bacteria join forces to ward off intruders and ensure that long fermentation can be accomplished without external contamination.

Although their research advanced our understanding of this particular microbial liaison, the honor of discovering the essential role of microorganisms themselves in all fermentation, which in reality is a decaying process, belongs to Louis Pasteur. His ingenious research in the mid-1800s led directly to the development of baker's cultured yeasts, primarily fast-acting *Saccharomyces cerevisiae*. As Tom Gumpel and others point out, it serves the needs of industrial bakers better than the nutritional needs of the consumers who buy their products. To home bakers, it's Fleischmann's. *S. cerevisiae* bears little in common with sourdough's cultures, which thrive at temperatures too cold for baker's yeasts.

Since Egyptians began leavening bread in about 1500 BCE—almost certainly by accident when yeasty brewery grain got mixed in with the emmer wheat flour they used—bakers employed leftover chunks of unbaked dough to hatch new batches of starter. The starter itself, like the caveman's cherished torch, passed down through generations, protected at all costs to keep fires lit, has acquired its own survival mythology. In winter gold-prospecting forty-niners often lived on sourdough and hung the starter from their neck against their chest in a small box to keep it warm and alive for the next loaf, as did Klondike Gold Rush miners. A noble effort but a misguided tactic: sourdough starters survive best in cold, not heat. When you take that San Francisco lactobacillus away from its home in the Bay Area, I've been asked, does it create the same starter in a different environment? No, it adjusts to the neighborhood. Environmental conditions change the blend of bacteria and yeast.

As you continue to refresh the starter in Brooklyn, for instance, "local bugs join the party," as King Arthur Flour baking director Jeffrey Hamelman puts it. After a month or so you will be whipping up a starter batch containing a companion *Lactobacillus brooklynensis*, whose flavor and microbial properties will lend it a unique Flatbush accent. For that reason a sourdough miche from Bien Cuit bakery in Cobble Hill offers a distinctively different taste and texture than one from the Acme Bread Company in Berkeley.

Fermentation scientists have shown that no matter where that bread is made, its lactic bacteria and primary yeast strain behave in the same symbiotic fashion, creating hyperactive live cultures that ferment wheat much as they convert milk to yogurt. Small amounts of ripe starter in a bowl with added flour and water produce a levain, or pre-ferment, where that microbial conversion slowly expands. The levain in time gets added to larger measures of flour and water and salt, and with a baker's astute assistance the process continues until the final dough is fully fermented—two to three days from star to finish.

Peter Reinhart, the dean of American bread writers, compares fermenting dough to making epoxy—the process, not the final result. Imagine the ripened levain with starter as one tube, a bowl of mixed final dough without it in another: you keep them separate until the optimum moment, a day or so after creating the levain, then you combine, thoroughly mix, add salt, bulk ferment, and proof (initiate a second rise) over another four to six hours. I spell that out because nature spells it out. You can't hurry love or sourdough microbes. Depending on where and how they are baked, the loaves will produce markedly different flavors, degrees of tanginess, and air-pocket sizes, but wherever that sourdough calls home, it will follow a similar regimen and also offer equivalent enriched taste and health benefits.

Informed Opinion

Back to science: if a little bit of knowledge is a dangerous thing, I was teetering on a narrow precipice. By now my research and personal experience combined to tempt me with suppositions that felt like reasonable conclusions. One was that the probiotic effect of eating naturally fermented sourdough, originating from its lactic acid bacteria, worked to bolster that community of microorganisms charged with keeping us healthy in body and mind, called our gut microbiome. Another convinced me that sourdough processing solved gluten's digestive issues for most non-celiacs. Both played into my pro-wheat, pro-sourdough bias, and I'd learned just enough from a lifetime of chasing down the truth to know that bias is a fur-lined trap, especially when it's unacknowledged. In journalism, as in science, when you seek out the opinion of impartial, qualified experts, you run the risk of dismantling your own beliefs and annulling the hard work of gathering the information that formed them. But the other option, to tell a lie, is really no option at all.

That conversation with myself led me to cereal microbiologist Michael Gaenzle, professor at the University of Alberta, Canada. Gaenzle is one of the scientific pioneers who have probed the microbial properties of sourdough—in many ways still a surprisingly new frontier when you consider that we've been eating naturally leavened wheat for three thousand years. He's published over 150 papers on cereal-associated lactic acid bacteria for use as starter cultures and probiotics in food. I knew what Marco Gobbetti had to say. I needed other informed opinions.

Gaenzle doesn't talk for long about his studies without bringing in prolamins and disulfide bonds. In fact, he's referred to them three times in the first few minute of our phone conversation. I feel like an atheist at a church service. Much of the language scientists use and the significance they attach to it orbit around me without ever making touchdown. I get the immediate basics from Gaenzle, I think, and that may be sufficient: disulfide bonds form bridges between the gliadin storage proteins, or prolamins, and in so doing, give them a compact structure that is difficult to break down by digestive enzymes. Sourdough's lactobacilli act as razors that sever those links and allow digestive enzymes to break down gluten proteins into small amino acid fragments, or peptides.

Gaenzle was on one of the first research teams that in 2004 checked into the relationship between gluten hydrolysis and sourdough fermentation. The team's study supplemented another in Italy in the same year that showed the use of selected lactobacilli and long fermentation in multigrain wheat sourdough to be "a novel tool for decreasing the level of gluten intolerance in humans."

What does all this mean in the simplest terms? I asked him. "Does sourdough processing break up most of the bad stuff or not?"

"Not for celiac sufferers," he said. "For them artisanal breads like that are just as toxic as commercial breads, the gluten reduction may be 5 percent at most."

"That's a small percent. Is it enough for most of the rest of us?"

"For anyone who's sensitive but not celiac, it can help. Imagine that you've got a tightly wound ball of string, and you unravel it. That's lactic bacteria pulling apart compact gluten proteins. We need more research before we can prove it definitively."

Which brought me to my next question. "We've got millions of people around the world now wondering if wheat is good or bad for them but no new reliable information; the last big study was four years ago. Where are the current ones we need?"

"It's true, there is a lot of public reaction and not a lot of good science," Gaenzle said. "The gluten-free phase is a relatively new phenomenon, and science is terribly slow. By the time we've written our proposal and trained our grad students, etcetera, and publish, you might as well add four or five years. But soon we'll start to see good science on what gluten sensitivity is and what could be the causes for it. I'm quite sure we will have good science, too, on what we need to do to prevent it."

In the meantime, he added, there is a lot of overreaction. Then he gave me a more panoramic view of the terrain. "What we will find, I think, is that wheat, like all plants, is not intended to be eaten." By which he meant that they only want us to spread their seeds. "Whatever the plant does, it aims to provide energy for the embryo, and we're eating the grain before it can grow."

"But that's true for all seeds that we eat, pumpkin, sesame, whatever."

Yes, said Gaenzle, but wheat especially contains an enzyme that can cause an allergic reaction; it's simply the plant's way of protecting itself from being eaten.

Does sourdough come into play here? I wondered.

"Very much! The little bit of the disulfide reduction and protein degradation you get from sourdough can be enough to deactivate that enzyme."

On the one hand, wheat yeasts produce amylase needed to break down complex sugars and facilitate digestion. On the other, in a self-protective mode, wheat kernels produce an inhibitor specifically designed to thwart that conversion. As Gaenzle pointed out, plants do not make it easy for us to invade and plunder unless the process forwards their propagation.

Wanted, Dead or Alive

Elsewhere this energetic microbiologist has posited an interesting theory, which is that sourdough cultures become so intimately bound up with us as a home or artisan baker and fermenter over time that, on a microbial level, the bread we make is tailor-made to support and nourish only us. As writer Katherine Czapp explains

Gaenzle's idea, "This 'home advantage' is an obvious traditional benefit conferred on newly married daughters whose mothers included a barrel of sourdough in the wedding dowry to start their new households—to ensure their daughters' health and vigor . . . and provide them extra strength in their new positions in life."

The idea of a customized microbial relationship between my bread and me steered the conversation from plant to gut—and to the various ways sourdough's lactic acid bacteria (LAB) improves and repairs the health of our microflora—or so I thought. A brief excursion provides relevant background:

The microbiome and probiotics—microorganisms like yogurt's acidophilus—are hot topics in health and wellness circles these days. Our systems are said to thrive on probiotics, and many believe—myself among them, for a time—that a prime source is sourdough's lactic acid bacteria. A Los Angeles artisan bread baker, Jack Bezian, has developed an ultra-long-fermented—we're talking up to a month—sourdough process, celebrated by his devoted customers as a delivery system for superpowered LAB, whether true or not. Those bacteria are known to repair gut wall damage created by prolonged antibiotic use and to help heal irritable bowel syndrome. Clinical studies now show that probiotic therapy is also effective in treating diarrhea and vaginal and urinary tract infections in women.

Until I looked into sourdough's therapeutic properties, my connection to probiotics, aside from eating yogurt and drinking kefir, consisted mostly of walking past bottles with unpronounceable names and unaffordable prices in the refrigerated sections of health food stores and Whole Foods. Lactobacillus, I learned, has long been hailed as one of the "friendly" bacteria that breaks down food, absorbs nutrients, and bolsters defense actions by gut cells against microbial mischief. In the first decade of the 1900s, Nobel Prize winner Elie

Metchnikoff discovered that lactic acid in particular boosts the immune system and maintains a functional digestive tract. He was so convinced of its therapeutic value that he drank a glass of sour milk every day. Glucose breaks down in our muscles during extreme exercise to produce the same lactic acid with beneficial results: it helps maintain your energy level as you push yourself. (Lactose, in milk, is a sugar and has no connection to lactic acid.)

More than a century later, we're still taking Elie's advice but with a better understanding of our gut microbiome's complexity. Someday we'll be able to monitor the internal processing of the food we eat as we eat it, organ by organ, and check our wristwatch interface for an immediate status report on digestive progress and microbial compatibility. Until then, we have to make do with a mash-up of science and intuitive body awareness. In that arena the most interesting research I came across forges a direct link between mind and microbiome.

Writing in the *American Psychological Association Journal*, Dr. Siri Carpenter summarizes recent rodent studies showing that the health of your gut influences emotional behavior, neural development, brain chemistry, and hormonal stress levels. In one project a strain of timid mice were given a cocktail of antibiotics, completely changing their behavior. They became bold and adventurous. When the antibiotics were removed, the mice reverted to their former cautious selves. "How could gut bacteria influence the brain and behavior so profoundly?" asks Carpenter. "One way, some studies indicate, is by co-opting the immune system itself, using immune cells and the chemicals they synthesize to send messages to the brain." But, she continues, some bacteria can induce behavioral changes even without triggering an immune response, suggesting that other channels of gut-brain communication must be at work.

You can understand why I was eager to check out sourdough's

powerhouse LAB with Michael Gaenzle—and how dispirited I was, at least temporarily, to learn that the baking oven's high heat kills off sourdough's bacteria before the bread is eaten. Bad news for my intuitive guess, based on personal, anecdotal experience.

I asked Gaenzle if in that case, aside from scissoring gluten molecules into digestible fragments, there were any health benefits to sourdough. "There are a couple of good leads on how sourdough does indeed improve health," he said. "Starch becomes less digestible, so the glycemic index goes down. There is fiber produced through one type of saccharides, mineral availability is increased by the degradation of phytates, and there are other important metabolic conversions."

"And lactic acid bacteria is not one of the reasons. From what you're telling me, there is nothing probiotic in sourdough."

"Well, it's a little more complicated. Not all of the benefits related to probiotic bacteria require viable cells, so it is entirely possible or even likely that material from dead cells in sourdough bread has beneficial effects. There is no data demonstrating this effect, though."

It's not simply the bacteria, Dr. W. Allan Walker told me. It's the acid as well. Walker, a professor in the Department of Nutrition at the Harvard School of Public Health, founded a research lab to study mucosal immunology. "The production of acid is good for health-promoting bacteria and bad for pathogens. There's a lot of evidence to suggest that the acid produced by lactobacillus may be one of its protective factors." Sourdough, in short, is at the very least prebiotic—a food source that helps beneficial gut bacteria to thrive.

What about those dead sourdough cells we carry around in our guts? I asked. How can they be beneficial?

"You don't necessarily have to have the organism in the food that the individual is ingesting. Food itself and its ingested products can facilitate the proliferation of these helpful bacteria. It could very well be that components of the digestive products of sourdough increase lactic acid bacteria as they ferment in the colon. Sourdough may well have health-promoting nutritional effects."

And that's science, I thought to myself. It traffics in the living attributes of dead cells and accommodates other messy uncertainties when most of us—myself, for one—struggle simply to ferret out trustworthy guidance that we can apply to our own highly unscientific daily lives. Science also seems to lag behind the curve or catapult way ahead of it. Artisan bread bakers, on the other hand, are entirely present tense. They have little choice—their customers return for more or go elsewhere based on today's bake. They know a lot about sourdough, these bakers, and almost none of what they know comes from research papers. The source of the information resides in their customers' taste buds, stomachs, and alimentary canals. That sort of anecdotal evidence surrounds sourdough like a warm blanket—a well-traveled, many-layered one.

For over a year I heard variants on the same story told to me by these bakers from Hawaii to Nova Scotia and from Melbourne to Scotland: word of mouth (literally) convinced their gluten-sensitive customers to risk trying sourdough. They reported back a symptom-free bread-eating experience, often to their surprise, and have now become regular sourdough purchasers.

Laycie Love's experiment with sourdough on the big island of Hawaii represents an extreme transition that captures their sense of elation and relief. She suffered from gastrointestinal problems her entire life, acute bowel inflammation as well as Ménière's disease, a vertigo disorder; in combination they sent her to the emergency ward six times in one month. Turning twenty-five, Love set out to take a proactive approach. She cut out gluten and put herself on a raw-food diet. At a farmer's market she met Steve Van Dermyden, owner of Oven & Butter Artisan Bakery in Captain Cook, directly west of Mauna Lea. Concerned about the possibility of suffering from Crohn's autoimmune disease, she was wary of trying his bread, even after he explained that his twenty-hour fermentation process seemed to reduce or eliminate gluten difficulties. "I remember taking just one bite," she said, "and I knew immediately that it was okay, because other breads would make my throat swell up." She waited thirty minutes and tried another bite, with no adverse reaction. "Having been under the assumption that I was never again going to be able to eat bread, the fact that I can regularly do that is a beautiful thing to me."

To Keith Cohen, who owns Orwasher's Bakery on New York's Upper East Side, Love's discovery sounds a familiar theme. "People I've spoken to with supposed gluten intolerances have had my rye bread and sourdough and spelt, all made with native yeasts, and they're fine." One of the city's oldest continuing bakery operations, Orwasher's has been turning out quality loaves for over a hundred years. In 2009 Cohen created a new line of artisan wine breads with a wine grape starter in collaboration with Channing Daughters Winery on Long Island. He is the kind of fanatic you want your baker to be; recently he spent close to a year in France studying with a world master to learn how to make the perfect baguette. He buys as much wheat as possible from New York growers, in part to help support the state's agricultural economy and in part to avail himself of freshness that regional live dough delivers to the company's baked goods.

Cohen stands in for the broad spectrum of artisan bakers I

talked with. He's opinionated, as most are, and not in the least concerned that anyone without celiac disease can tolerate his sourdoughs, now that he's observed his customers' reactions over the years. He's not waiting for the scientific community to play catch-up. "I am a firm believer that bread made the way we do it is perfectly fine for you. Modern-day bread is the cause of gluten intolerance. It's taken forty years for the chicken to come home to roost."

If Cohen's sourdough customers knew they were eating dead lactic acid bacteria that may still oddly be probiotic, or at least prebiotic, would it matter? Probably not. Or if they learned that sourdough releases bound minerals and makes them more bioavailable? Maybe. But like the rest of us, it's safe to say that for them, health benefits rank behind eating pleasure. Taste and texture matter first and foremost. Long-fermented sourdough shows off wheat's sass and substance in ways that highlight the harmonious contradictions of spunky acid and caramelized grain sugar. It *feels* healthy. As Cohen pointed out to me, sourdough takes its rightful place among the holy trinity of the fermentations—bread, cheese, and wine: "the things we live for," as he succinctly summarizes their rightful place.

Who could disagree? Many of us, according to Bay State Milling VP Mike Pate—at least, about sourdough. "It's a shame that more people don't have a taste for it," he said. "But let's be honest. Lactobacillus has a pH of 3.4; it's noticeably acidic and not everybody's cup of tea. There's no way sourdough will ever dominate the mainstream, but as we see more and more of these bakery-cafés come along, I think you'll see it continue to grow."

The local artisans whose baked goods are sold in those cafés are wheat consumers, too. Among the things that they have in common is a fixation on quality flour—as in fresh, possibly local, most likely stone-ground, maybe oxidized to a degree if white for better performance but not roller-milled to dust. To Dan Barber, chef and co-owner of the Blue Hill restaurant, commodity flour arrives "dead." Flour alive with enzymes—organic rye, in particular—delivers the microbial agents that most reliably kick off sourdough starters.

"I've been banging my fist on the table about sourdough *forever*," Panera's head baker, Tom Gumpel, said. "Seventeen years ago, when I was dean of the Culinary Institute of America, I was hosting a husband and wife who were true celiacs and were starting the Celiac Foundation. They wanted to get the word out, long before anyone in this country was talking about gluten. We're at dinner one night and this kid drops a huge breadbasket right in the middle of the table. We all laugh and I said to the kid, a student, 'Hey, do me a favor, take that away.' But as he reached for it the husband said, 'Hold on one second. Is there any sourdough in that basket?' I asked him why. He said, 'I can eat sourdough and have no autoimmune response.' It was like a *barbell* hit me in the head. I thought, Of *course*! With pre-consumption of carbohydrates, proteins being broken down, and all the enzymatic activity, long fermentation takes that issue out of the equation."

Gumpel calls his goals for Panera "aspirational": to transform the traditional forms of bread we all eat—sandwich slices, for instance—into whole, healthful, naturally leavened products. For Gumpel, the rewards are worth the effort.

And So It Goes

If only the things we love to eat loved us back in return. Unrequited love's a bore, as Rodgers and Hart reminded us. In this scenario long fermentation, soaking, and sprouting are nature's matchmakers; they make no promise of living happily ever after, but they introduce grain to gut in its most desirable, compatible, and efficacious form and leave the rest to natural attraction.

Although we're not ruminants equipped to eat grass, we are smart enough to learn from our surroundings. We see how living things beneficially degrade in nature and we mimic that behavior by corralling and utilizing two fundamental allies, air and water. Still, matchmaking takes time, and the time it takes is both a blessing and curse. Soaking, sprouting, and long fermentation offer us a chance to pay attention to the rhythms of nature, a slow and steady beat when enzymatic conversions are at play. The downside for some is that in the frenzied pace of contemporary life, waiting is stressful. Our digestive systems, on the other hand, are not time-sensitive. They function by an independent internal clock. What matters is that they receive the rewards of us acting as the responsible tenant of our own body rather than as an absentee owner. When offered grain with all of its nutritive components left intact, in a state that helps us consume it without difficulty or danger, that system more often than not cooperates and flourishes.

It's the part of the story that somehow got left out in the barrage of invective against wheat, and only with that part included is there a complete and true story to tell.

The Bottom Line

The three principles I put forward in these pages—white's not right, long's not wrong, and whole takes no toll—are intended as a quick reminder when out in the world making your way along a grocery store aisle or standing in a bakery line, but not as the eleventh through thirteenth commandments. In more extended form, they're meant to help keep in mind that refined white flour is bad for you, that lomg fermented sourdoughs are good for you, and that 100 percent whole wheat is beneficial, not injurious.

If you want to cheat occasionally, the medical experts I talked with advise you to do just that—make it occasional, as in once a week, not every other day. Based on my research experience, I'd also strongly urge you to go exploring. Among the many things I now know that I didn't when I started my research is that the universe of ancient grains delivers unexpected gifts. I'd never until now really spent time with any of them. They may make practical sense for any non-celiac with an extreme sensitivity to modern wheat. Einkorn is easier to digest than today's wheat, and, ten thousand years later, it still makes delicious breads and cookies.

When I began my exploration I knew only that I enjoyed sourdough bread, but nothing about its microbial health and digestive advantages. Unfortunately, the substantial benefits of long fermentation and sprouting, I discovered, have not adequately been addressed by researchers in our country. That appears to be directly linked to a lack of sufficient funding for clinical studies. At a time when gluten and carbohydrate issues occupy so much pubic attention, I find that puzzling and disheartening.

Simply put, if the nation's large cereal companies, such as General Mills, choose to deal with attacks on wheat by chasing a gluten-free trend that offers zero nutrition, that's a business strategy. But to their discredit, in my view, they have also made no attempt to bring long fermentation to the mainstream consumer at an affordable cost, or to fund research in that area. "Considering how many people in the US are having problems tolerating specific foods and the potential negative health consequences, it's amazing how little interest there is in funding research to understand why this is happening to us," microbiota researcher Justin Sonnenburg observes.

Clinical studies in Europe, particularly in Italy, provide solid evidence that naturally fermented dough can play a crucial part in delivering the nutrients and fiber of whole wheat while mitigating the problems associated with gluten.

I'm well aware that my own experience as a consumer of artisan sourdoughs is a privilege, one that would not be affordable if I were buying bread or other baked goods to feed a large family on a tight budget. Long-fermented products cost more to make and to buy. Still, if there proved to be a viable market for whole-wheat sourdoughs at a reasonable price point, I suspect the ingenuity of these industrial cereal companies would meet the challenge. At present we appear to be penalizing less affluent families by limiting their access to the most healthful wheat products and, by doing so, fostering rampant obesity. Hasn't the time come for companies that supply our nation with empty white-flour calories by way of refined flour to step up and take a stand for 100 percent whole-grain nutrition? Their shortcuts may save money, but at a cost to our health and welfare that is incalculable. We all deserve better treatment, independent of family income. The time has arrived.

For ten thousand years bread has been the edible contract that binds speaker to listener. It's as close as we come to swapping and swallowing the same source of nourishment as a pledge of mutual fidelity. That doesn't yet take into account the religious sacramental significance of water mixed into wheat flour. Priests for millennia have placed wafers of grain representing the body of Christ on the tongues of Roman Catholic congregants (those, at any rate, who do not today insist on gluten-free substitutes). Observant Jews recite the *Ha-motzi* blessing over two raised loaves of freshly baked challah every Friday night to honor the Sabbath. Strip references to bread and wheat out of the Old and New Testaments and you come away with two thin books. Throwing bread, a gift from Allah, into the trash is unethical in Islam.

Given that, I wasn't surprised to discover that the word *companion* has its Latin roots in breaking bread together. Bread imparts a sense of trust in elemental basics—especially the notion that in the company of such an honest food, honest people share honest truths. For most of us, I think, wheat-based baked goods, from mouthwatering baguette to warm yeasty French country loaf, merge private enjoyment with social bonding.

Good health, to me, is what good bread is all about, both mental and physical. It comes from wheat grown and nurtured in harmony with nature's cycles—then, now, and long into the future.

If I've done anything to return you to that abandoned pleasure safe and sound, I consider this project well worth all my time and attention, and hopefully yours, too.

Acknowledgments

I had the title for *Grain of Truth* before I had any idea of how to get where I wanted to go, which was simply to tell a more balanced, less sensational story about wheat than I kept bumping into online and in print.

Real nourishing and delicious bread did not seem to be getting a fair hearing, but if it, along with all other wheat products, turned out to be as bad for us as the anti-gluten movement claimed, so be it—I decided to investigate.

More than eighteen months, a hundred-plus interviews, and a few thousand miles later, I owe my deepest gratitude to everyone whose generosity with their time and knowledge made that possible. My grasp of science I quickly realized would be mightily tested; Kevin Comerford helped me to glean useful information from numerous abstruse research papers. Luckily, the microbiologists who came to my rescue in the United States and Italy demonstrated considerable patience in explaining the workings of our gut microbiome and the fermentation shenanigans of sourdough, as did the agricultural scientists in illuminating genetics. All insights are theirs. Any mistakes are entirely mine.

Michael Gaenzle at the University of Alberta, one of the leading experts on lactic acid bacteria, answered dozens of questions over several months and contributed his invaluabe insights. Marco Gobbetti at the University of Bari in Italy, who has also participated in numerous studies on long fermentation, shared his intimate knowledge, as did Dr. Harold (Dusty) Dowse, a scientist and avid sourdough baker at the University of Maine. America's dean of bread making, Peter Reinhart, a good guy all around—and fabulous bread and pizza magician—led me to him. Dr. W. Allan Walker at Harvard walked me through the narrow straits dividing pre- and probiotics. Dr. Peter Gibson in Melbourne gave me a rundown on Fodmaps and explained how a reaction can be confused with gluten sensitivity. Drs. Alessio Fasano and Stefano Guandalini, two of our most respected celiac disease specialists, took time to share their updated findings with me.

David Killilea at the Oakland Children's Hospital walked me through the role of long fermentation in freeing up locked minerals in flour, as well as the vast nutritional differences between "whole"—51 percent—and 100 percent whole wheat. Dr. Ayala Laufer-Cahana reminded me that, as Henry Miller observed, we often give our bodies orders that make no sense. Katherine Czapp directed me to an essay she wrote on her father's bout with celiac disease, and his struggle to restore his health, that brought home the wisdom of the body.

Whenever I got in trouble on that subject, usually by assuming I knew something I hadn't fully understood, I often turned to nutritionist Julie Miller Jones. Having her looking over my shoulder (in spirit) gave me an enormous boost of confidence and saved me from making innumerable errors. My special thanks to her. For studies on the benefit of 100 percent whole wheat I thank Len Marquart, a professor of food science at the University of Minnesota and president of the Grains for Health Foundation, for pointing me in the right direction. Nutrition experts David R. Jacobs and Monica Spiller and Cynthia Harriman at oldways.com, among others, amplified my knowledge. Joe Vanderliet and Keith and Nicky Giusto gave me a quick but intense education in milling. All three devote themselves to bringing out the best in a wheat kernel.

Brian Walker at Horizon made it possible to get a firsthand look at industrial milling and baking. He made an extra effort to give me access to the way wheat arrives on our table and at fast-food chains today, which I deeply appreciate.

Then, too, there was wheat in the field to learn all about. Brad Seabourn and Stan Cox and Brett Carver—all located near or in the Grain Belt—pitched in with their understanding of the wheat farming community, the chemistry of the wheat seed, and more. Bob Graybosch at the USDA in Lincoln, Nebraska, sent illustrations of the gluten protein and answered a slew of questions about gluten with equanimity and clarity, both deeply appreciated. Helpful, too, was Donald Kasarda. Geneticist Steve Lyon at Washington State showed me how to crossbreed. And to Steve Jones, director of the WSU Research Center, I owe thanks for making clear every difference between commodity and local heritage wheat as a crop and as a life's calling. My thanks, too, to Wendy Hebb, program director for the Kneading Conference—since renamed the Grain Gathering—who graciously made it possible for me to attend that splendid event. Maggie Beidelman shared contacts she made for her delightful documentary, *The Trouble with Bread*, which is sure worth seeking out.

For insights into heritage and ancient grains, my thanks go to

Carla Bartolucci at Jovial Foods and to Eli Rogosa. For a historical lesson on grain and wheat and bread and their role in our evolution, thanks to Clifford Wright, William Rubel, and Darra Goldstein. For letting me tag along to public school, Erik Finnerty at Fat Cat and Janice Cooper at the California Wheat Commission, a friend of the project and a fellow Ponsford pizza-lover. Thanks, too, to Paul Muller at Full Belly Farms in the Capay Valley of Northern California. Muller brought me into his organic heritage wheat fields and left me with hope for trusting small, dedicated farmers like him to preserve our planet's cherished resources. To Bob Klein at Community Grains, a special salute for introducing me to the exploding West Coast artisanal wheat movement and for allowing me to snoop around in his "Grain Trust" at will. In New York, June Russell at GrowNYC, in charge of the farmer's market grain contingent, put me in touch with many of New York's local wheat gurus including Don Lewis at Wild Hive in the Hudson Valley, the guys at Sfoglini, and Zach Golper, who arranged for me to be an apprentice baker for a day at Bien Cuit, his fabulous Brooklyn bakery. And while on the subject of bakers, my thanks to Craig Ponsford, Steve Sullivan at Acme Bread Company, Eduardo Morell at Morell's Bread in Berkeley, Steven Van Dermyden at Hawaii's Oven & Butter and to Tom Gumpel at Panera, who is determined to cross the dividing line between mainstream and artisanal heritage wheat—a task well suited to Gumpel's cyclonic energy and determination. For his Italian pasta insights, my thanks to Andrew Curry.

One of the first friends of this project, Michael Pollan, generously shared his sources from *Cooked* and encouraged me at the earliest stage. "There's much more about wheat still to be told," he said, and he was right. My editor, Wendy Wolf, and I easily picked up a dialogue we started years back on my first book with her, and when it came down to final editing I was reminded once again of my good fortune. If writing is music, Wendy is the deft conductor who, with a tiny flick of the baton, keeps all of the instruments in perfect synchronization, and always with a sense of humor. I'm grateful as well to Caroline Sutton for stepping up to green-light the project. Good friends Tony Cook, Joan Barnes, and Michael Coffino kept me entertained and diverted through difficult passages, devoured my sourdoughs as an act of solidarity, and offered valuable counsel whenever summoned.

My best friend and most trusted ally of all, I am deeply grateful to report, is my wife, Bonnie, who reads every word and brings all of her professional and intuitive wisdom to the task. She has an unerring ear for truth, an admirable impatience for cant, and a belief in me that after all these years I now realize is unshakable. Not a word in this book went out into the world without first passing through her checkpoint. I can't imagine writing or living without her, or our wonderful grown offspring, Josh, Omri, and Yael, their mates Jackie and Eli, and their rambunctious, inquisitive kids who give us no choice but to be ready to crawl on the floor or play hide-and-seek at a moment's notice. They remind us not to take ourselves too seriously, which may be the greatest gift of all.

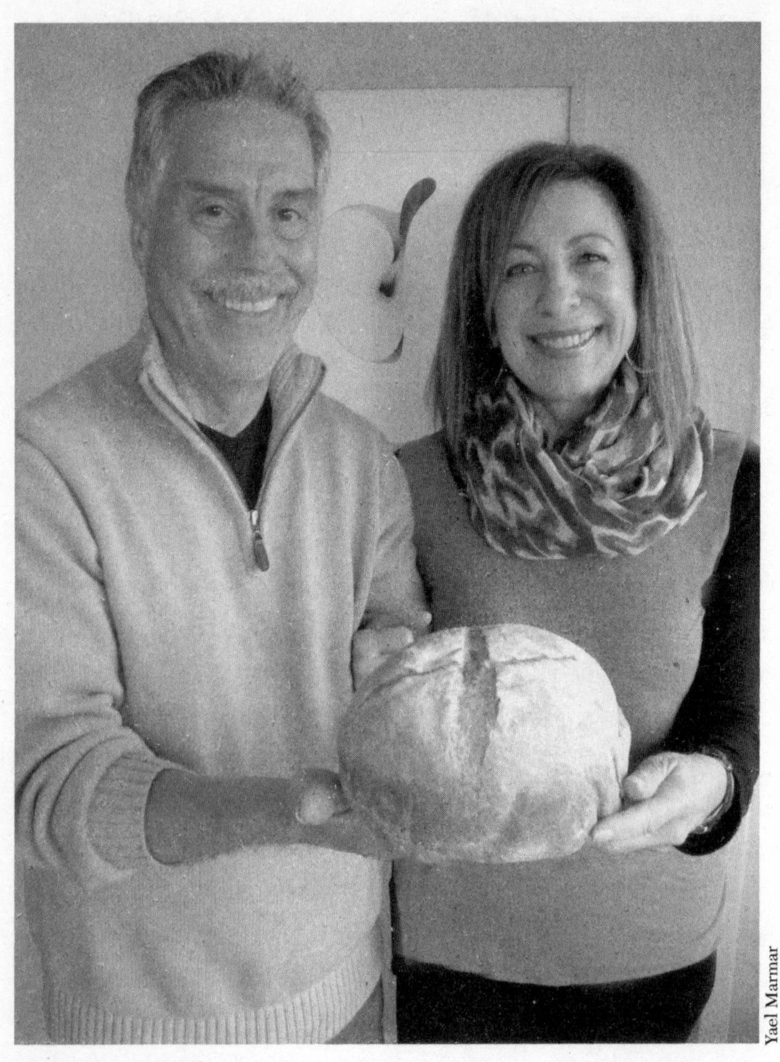
Yael Marmar

The author and his wife, Bonnie Trust Dahan,
with a loaf of still-warm sourdough straight from the oven.

Appendix A

FINAL FIVE WHOLE-WHEAT SOURDOUGH BREAD RECIPE

I've always been something of an improviser around the kitchen, tossing in a smidgen of this herb or that spice by the measurement of my palm, more or less equal to a teaspoon when cupped and expanding to a tablespoon when opened.

That works fine for soup ingredients and such, but not for bread, whose fate depends on a more scrupulous approach when weighing out liquids and solids, all by grams. Once I discovered that accuracy does not intrude on invention, and that in fact it ensures more reliable results, I traded in my palm for implements that provide exact quantities, and made a $20 investment in an EatSmart digital baker's kitchen scale that measures in grams, ounces, pounds, and kilograms.

Bread recipes are called formulas in the industry, I realized, because they function most effectively when bakers hew to precise protocols, from liquid volume to oven temperature. To eliminate any measurement guesswork, somebody way back invented baker's math.

"Baker's math," George De Pasquale, owner of Essential Baking in Seattle, told us in a Kneading Conference hands-on session, "is the bones of bread making, and it's important to understand because as a baker your real job is fermenting, or growing a civilization of microbes. Everything about your bread dough is impacting the way those microbes grow."

By basing proportions of all ingredients by percentage relative to the total weight of flour, which is always expressed as 100 percent, baker's math, calculated in grams, removes all confusions that develop from converting liquid ounces to solid ounces, and so forth. If the formula calls for 60 percent hydration and 400 grams of flour (100 percent), you add 240 grams of water to make the dough, no more or less, and so it goes.

Final Five Sourdough Recipe

Although my wife, Bonnie, dropped the last five pounds she could never before shed by eating a slice or two of my Final Five bread just about every day, none of the ingredients call for diet-friendly substitutes. Like any other naturally leavened sourdough, this recipe comes down to water + flour + salt + nature + heat. It requires about an hour of my time stretched over two or three days. Most of the work is done by the dough itself as it ferments and glutenizes while I'm sleeping, writing, running, or otherwise engaged. I pop in occasionally to blend, stir, mold, proof, and bake.

Active Time: 45 to 60 minutes

Total Time: 5 to 8 Days

Tip #1: Clean up as you proceed. Wet dough sticks and hardens as it dries. Use a lot of water and a little soap on bowls and equipment, and just let things soak if you can't get to them quickly.

Starter

I suggest that you do what I did, surround yourself with experts. Jeffrey Hamelman's instructions on the King Arthur Flour website combine photos of every starter stage with clear instructions. Hamelman, King Arthur's head baker, offers his own spin on Peter Reinhart's starter recipe in *The Bread Baker's Apprentice*. Go to the website for King Arthur and select "blog" from the top menu. Once there, type "Creating Your Own Sourdough" in the search field. A step-by-step guide will direct you to producing a bubbling starter in about a week. If you screw up, and the concoction smells like wet socks or sour booze, toss it out and start again. Another option, in addition to hundreds of online posts at Breadtopia, The Fresh Loaf, and elsewhere, is Andrew Whitley's *Bread Matters* for a rye starter. All contain excellent starter recipes. A third option is to send away for a premade starter on Amazon, a package of granules that you activate at home. Expose any starter to plenty of air and stir twice a day. The microbes thrive on oxygen. The mix should be about as thick as pancake batter.

Tip #2: Use organic whole-grain wheat or rye at the beginning of the process, not all-purpose flour. Both contain more nutrients and sourdough-friendly microorganisms.

Tip #3. Use filtered water only. Chlorinated water kills useful bacteria.

Making the Levain

About 12 to 16 hours before you plan to bake the bread, add ¼ cup (56 grams) of your fermented starter to ½ cup (140 grams) of filtered (non-chlorinated) lukewarm water and 100 grams each of organic all-purpose and whole-wheat flour. Stir vigorously, cover, and set aside overnight in a warm (75°F) place. It should rise as it ferments and a dollop of it should float in a glass of water.

Tip #4: You can set the nonmetallic bowl down on a plant propagator on top of a folded towel to warm it in a cool kitchen during winter months.

Mixing the Dough

After experimenting—that is, borrowing and adjusting master-baker formulas—I arrived at multigrain bread that is dense and filling but not heavy and brick-like. I like assertive sourness countered by a hint of sweetness, so I add a tablespoon of honey. To create the final organic dough, I mix 600 grams of whole wheat with 350 grams of all-purpose flour, 250 grams of rye, the optional honey, 760 grams of water, and 25 grams of sea salt. Many bakers sieve the whole-wheat flour to sift out bran flakes that can puncture the air holes. I do and don't, based on time constraints. The differences for me are minimal.

Add the levain to the dough. Because you are making bread with a majority of whole-wheat flour, it will not respond by ballooning as robustly as white-flour, high-gluten breads do. To assist the rise, some bakers add 3 to 4 grams of instant yeast to the mix. Hold off on adding the salt, which inhibits gluten activation. To mix by hand, put on an apron, wash your hands, roll up your sleeves, and dig in. You'll find the dough a wet, sticky mess at first, but as you continue to churn it—imagine your hands are rotating bicycle pedals—you'll find that the pulling and stretching begins to build an internal structure that enables the dough, in time, to support itself and, in effect, develop tensile strength.

Bakers recommend about 500 or so vigorous strokes. That takes anywhere from 12 to 15 minutes. Insert rest breaks. I find the process to be strenuous—your arms feel it— and meditative at the same time, also informative. As you feel the dough transform, you learn to gauge its degree of completion.

Stand mixers offer a second option. I eventually bought a KitchenAid Pro and sometimes use the hook attachment for the first part of the blending at the lowest speed for 3 minutes, then after a 30-minute rest, at Position 2 for another 3 minutes or until it cleans the bowl. I continue to mix by hand until I can feel that it is ready. You literally want to get in touch with your dough. Either way, let it sit for 20 to 30 minutes before you stir in the salt—and optionally 40 grams of water if too dense.

Autolyze is the baker's term for these critical rest periods. It enables the enzymes in flour—amylase and protease—to begin to break down the starch and gluten protein and absorb moisture. Long fermentation techniques allow for the cleaving of bulky gluten molecules, but you do not reduce their ability to provide elasticity and extensibility.

Bulk Ferment

Once the salt is added, I transfer the dough to a large bowl, and use a no-knead process to create smooth, buoyant dough. Every 40 to 45 minutes or so I reach in with a wet hand, grip the bottom of the mix, pull up high, then fold gently on top before turning the dough 45 degrees and repeating the exercise. Over five or six sessions, spread over 3 hours, the dough becomes increasingly more self-reliant.

Dividing and Shaping

First, I flour a work surface and turn the dough out; then I divide it into two equal units using a plastic dough scraper. Using the heel of my palm I stretch each out into a rectangle, fold and stretch again a few times, with a bowl of flour nearby to add to my hands as needed. The dough is moist yet not sticky. In time I fold the rectangle, first overlapping one end about one third of the way down, then bringing in each of its edges like an envelope at 45 degrees to create a vertical central line. Once the bottom two edges of the rectangle are turned in the same manner, the top section is rolled all the way to the end. I work this fat cylinder back and forth and cup its edges as I turn it to form a globe.

After working on that for a month or so I began to get the hang of it, which is to pull down slightly on the surface with the side of the hand as I turn, smoothing and making taut that surface "skin" of the dough. Master bakers like Chad Robertson make this a balletic movement, a muscular dance. There are no doubt YouTubes on the technique, but practice alone enabled me to become more proficient. No need to be intimidated: the bread is not being offered for sale on a retail shelf; if its surface is slightly bumpy, so be it.

When both globes are shaped, I cover for 30 minutes with a towel.

Proofing

The second fermentation period, when the globes rise again for a few hours, is called proofing because it proves that the bread is in fact ready to bake. (You can also refrigerate these shaped loaves to retard fermentation after they proof, and bake the following day. The acetic, souring acid in sourdough becomes more assertive at a colder temperature. Warm to room temperature before baking.) To proof, dust two bowls with flour, as well as the globes, and then flip each upside down—you'll see a bottom seam—into a bowl. I use wicker-proofing bowls that I eventually purchased for this stage, but any large bowls will do. Cover and let stand. Whitley uses large tented plastic bags as coverings to keep in the moisture.

Baking

Place Dutch oven in the oven with its lid on, and preheat to 500°F for 30 or more minutes. Carefully remove, set down the lid, and flip the proofing bowl so that the globe drops into the bottom of the Dutch oven and lands on its seam side. Dough is forgiving. If you don't drop it straight in, it will re-form while baking, no worries. Score the top of the dough with a razor or serrated knife to allow gas to escape, cover, and bake at 460°F for 20 to 25 minutes. Remove the Dutch oven, take off the lid, and bake uncovered at 430°F for another 25 minutes.

Tip #5: Line bottom of Dutch oven with parchment paper to prevent dough from sticking.

These times are somewhat arbitrary, since all ovens perform differently. If you own a meat thermometer, use it. You want to remove the bread when the internal temperature reaches 200°F, not before. A hollow drum sound when you tap on the bottom also indicates that it is done. A reddish, foxy crust just on the verge of darkening to a deep brown is what you're after. Set on a rack, and resist eating it until it cools; this takes a few hours. It gets better with age over the first few days and stays fresh for a week or more. I enjoy the layered fig-like richness of the whole wheat, balanced by the tanginess of the acids, and Bonnie and I don't seem to tire of it.

Still, once in a while for variety I add pumpkin seeds, or I reverse the proportions of rye and white and add caraway seeds. While the sourdough process does not by itself add nutritional value to the white flour, it slows down the rate of glucose absorption in the bloodstream and improves the bread's texture. If you eliminate white flour entirely, you'll achieve a perfectly edible, quite dense loaf with little rise.

Baking two at once makes good sense as a baker based on economies of scale, but what to do with the second loaf? Freeze it. Once cooled, wrap it in plastic, then in aluminum foil. Defrost overnight when ready, heat the oven to 350°F, insert the loaf for 10 minutes, cool for at least an hour, and eat. It retains all of its flavor and texture.

Appendix B

LOCAL ORGANIC GRAIN AND FLOUR SOURCES*

Heirloom wheat grain varieties, some ancient, sometimes show up on grocery store shelves, but rarely are those products locally grown. These regional producers offer a fresh alternative. Websites are listed for mills that sell flour directly to consumers. I list these at www.stephenyafa.com as well under "Resources."

NEW ENGLAND

Aurora Mills and Farm also grows and mills only Maine grains.

Green Mountain Flour in Vermont produces stone-ground flours, cracked grains, porridges, and mixes that include wheat, spelt, rye, and triticale.

King Arthur Flour, Vermont-based and founded in 1790, proves that a large milling company can maintain high quality in its product selection and a true sense of community. Its website offers e-commerce, education, instruction, tips, and techniques in its blog section. Order at www. kingarthurflour.com.

*This listing is my expanded and revised version of the original www.culinate.com sidebar to an article, "Flour to the People," written by Amy Halloran, published October 17, 2013.

Maine Grains, located at Somerset Grist Mill—a former county jail—stone-grounds locally grown and sourced, non-pesticide grains. Online ordering "coming soon" at www.mainegrains.com/products.

Pioneer Valley Heritage Grain CSA in western Massachusetts directly connects farmers and customers.

Wheatberry Bakery, owned by Ben and Adrie Lester, helped create the Pioneer Valley CSA and garnered a USDA grant for sustainable community development.

NEW YORK

Farmer Ground Flour is stone-milled by Greg Mol from Thor Oechsner's local, organic hard red winter and spring wheats, including fabled Warthog in the Finger Lakes region.

North Country Farms uses two granite stones to produce flours and mixes from locally grown grains. Kevin Richardson runs the operation.

Wild Hive's pioneering Don Lewis stone-mills the organic grains he has revived in the Hudson Valley.

MID-ATLANTIC

Annville Mill, in Pennsylvania, mills organic pastry flour sourced locally.

MIDWEST

Great River Organic Milling, in Wisconsin, employs two great granite wheels and offers sixteen whole-grain single-source flours and blends. Order on Amazon.

Heartland Mill stone-grinds organic Turkey Red in the High Plains of west Kansas. Order at www.heartlandmill.com.

Lonesome Stone Milling is a stone mill for organic grains in Wisconsin. Order at www.lonesomestonemilling.com.

Windmill Flour uses an actual Dutch windmill to mill Michigan wheat.

SOUTH

Anson Mills is where Glenn Roberts runs an ambitious and influential local-grain program in South Carolina, where he focuses on heirloom antebellum varieties. Order at www.ansonmills.com/products.html.

Carolina Ground stone-grinds North Carolina grains. Order at carolinaground.com/flourshop/.

WEST

Bluebird Grain Farms, also in Washington State, offers certified organic heirloom grains from plow to package, including ancient emmer, or farro. Order at www.bluebirdgrainfarms.com/retail-products.html.

Camas Country Mill in Oregon, owned by Tom Hunton, uses a Danish stone-mill system to make flours from grains grown in Oregon's Willamette Valley.

Central Milling, in Petaluma, owned by Keith and Nicky Giusto, is one of the nation's largest and most reliable stone-ground millers of organic flour, providing Whole Foods and other specialty retailers with private label products from wheat grown mostly in Utah. It also sells directly to the public from its website. Highly recommended. Order at http://centralmilling.com/collections/all.

Community Grains, owned by Bob Klein, markets Joseph's Best organic whole-wheat flour under its own label. It is the only direct-to-consumer source. Order its range of local-grain products at www.communitygrains.com.

Fairhaven Organic Flour Mill in western Washington State, owned by Kevin and Matsuko Christenson. The mill offers a variety of local organic grains.

CANADA

One Degree Organic Foods, in Vancouver, sells a variety of heritage grains such as Red Fife grown by small organic farmers from Saskatchewan, Canada, to Germany to Java, including sprouted whole wheat. You can't order direct, but a map of the United States on the site directs you to retailers in your area that carry One Degree's products. Visit https://www.onedegreeorganics.com.

Appendix C

ANCIENT AND HERITAGE GRAIN AND FLOUR SOURCES

Here is a small sampling of ancient grain growers and millers. Be aware that the term *farro* can create confusion. It commonly refers to emmer, but it is also used by some millers to describe einkorn and spelt as well, since farro is the Italian word for all three ancient hulled wheats. Order directly from websites.

Bluebird Grain Farms grows an abundance of emmer. See above. It also produces "einka farro"—whole grain einkorn flour. Visit www.bluebirdgrainfarms.com.

Cayuga Pure Organics in upstate New York is one of the few growers of emmer—better known as farro—in the United States. Visit www.cporganics.com.

Einkorn.com, Teton, Idaho. Jade Doyle grows more einkorn than anyone in the country, about 150,000 pounds annually on 150 acres. He sells its berries and will soon mill and sell high-nutritional einkorn flour directly to consumers. Einkorn, says Doyle, makes by far the fastest, best sourdough starter of any wheat.

Hayden Flour Mills in Tempe, Arizona, owned by Jeff Zimmerman, grows and stone-grinds white Sonora whole-wheat flour among other heritage grains including farro and sells them on his online store. Visit www.haydenflourmills.com.

Heritage Grain Conservancy in Colrain, Massachusetts, under Eli Rogosa's leadership, operates a farm where she and her staff grow and sell ancient einkorn as well as heritage varieties including Black Winter Emmer. Visit www.growseed.org.

Jovial Foods, located in Connecticut, produces a wide range of einkorn and other artisanal products from small organic growers in Italy. Visit www.jovialfoods.com.

Kamut is the trademarked brand name for khorasan wheat, a heritage tetraploid wheat subspecies high in the antioxidant selenium. Bob Quinn offers a complete history and much more, including product and source information in six languages at www.kamut.com.

Small Valley Milling in central Pennsylvania, operated by Elaine and Joel Steigman, mills organic spelt, the third ancient hulled grain. Visit www.smallvalleymilling.com.

Notes

Chapter One

11 **a *New Yorker* article:** Michael Specter, "Against the Grain," *New Yorker*, November 3, 2014.

20 **"cure this condition":** Julie M. Miller, "*Wheat Belly*—An Analysis of Selected Statements and Basic Theses from the Book," *Cereal Foods World*, July/August 2012, 177–89.

20 **"opiate drugs bind":** William Davis, *Wheat Belly* (New York: Rodale, 2011), 49.

20 **fullness, not hunger:** C. Zioudrou et al., "Opiod Peptide Derived from Food Proteins: The Exorphins," *Journal of Biological Chemistry* 254 (1979): 2446–49.

21 **answer: no and no:** Fred J. P. H. Brouns, et al., "Does Wheat Make Us Fat or Sick?," *Journal of Cereal Science* 58 (2013): 208–15. A comprehensive and persuasive study, dense with relevant references and thoroughly researched.

23 **"destroying your brain":** David Perlmutter with Kristin Loberg, *Grain Brain: The Surprising Truth About Wheat, Carbs, and Sugar—Your Brain's Silent Killers* (New York: Little, Brown, and Company, 2013), 4.

24 **"get a scapegoat; it's classic":** James Jamblin, "This Is Your Brain on Gluten," *Atlantic*, December 12, 2013, at www.theatlantic.com/health/archive/2013/12/this-is-your-brain-on-gluten/282550/.

Chapter Two

29 **specific genetic biomarkers:** The genetic disposition involves particular versions—DQ2 or DQ8—of a cellular receptor called the human leukocyte antigen (HLA), according to Dr. Alessio

Fasano, director of Mass General's Celiac Research Center in Boston.

31 **gluten just fine:** Moises Velasquez-Manoff, "Who Has the Guts for Gluten?" *New York Times*, February 23, 2013, at www.nytimes.com/2013/02/24/opinion/sunday/what-really-causes-celiac-disease.html?pagewanted=all.

32 **or microbial imbalance:** Anthony Samsel and Stephanie Seneff, "Glyphosate, Pathways to Modern Diseases II: Celiac Sprue and Gluten Intolerance," *Interdisciplinary Toxicology*, December 2013, 159–84.

33 **developed more tolerance:** http://www.pbs.org/wgbh/evolution/library/10/4/l_104_07.html.

33 **"Guts for Gluten":** http://www.nytimes.com/2013/02/24/opinion/sunday/what-really-causes-celiac-disease.html?pagewanted=all.

36 **A large Italian study:** Umberto Volta et al., "An Italian Prospective Multicenter Survey on Patients Suspected of Having Non-Celiac Gluten Sensitivity," Biomedcentral.com, May 23, 2014, at http://biomedcentral.com/1741-7015/12/85.

Chapter Three

39 **"that leads to it":** Tocqueville is quoted in Harold McGee, *On Food and Cooking* (New York: Scribner's, 1984), 519. No one I've read comes close to McGee as an authority on the science and culture of food. He is compulsively readable even when the text veers into the microbial universe where general readers fear to tread. McGee seems to know everything worth knowing about all foods and beverages. In the best tradition of an adventure guide, he pauses to point out smells, sights, and even sounds of interest. For more on Sylvester Graham, seek out Aaron Bobrow-Strain, *White Bread: A Social History of the Store-Bought Loaf* (Boston: Beacon Press, 2012). In it Bobrow-Strain provides a well-researched portrait of this conflicted man.

44 **most of society:** Michael Specter, "Against the Grain," *New Yorker*, November 3, 2014.

46 **movement took flight:** Vanessa Gregory, "Winning Without Wheat," *Men's Journal*, March 2010, 1–2. Aaron Bobrow-Strain in *White Bread: A Social History of the Store-Bought Loaf* deserves full credit for the investigative journalism linking pro-athlete performance to the rise of gluten-free in the public's awareness. Lim is the primary force behind the change from wheat to white rice, although 50 percent more rice is needed to achieve the same amount of glycogen muscle storage as wheat.

49 **"all of human evolution":** David Perlmutter with Kristin Loberg, *Grain Brain: The Surprising Truth About Wheat, Carbs, and Sugar—Your Brain's Silent Killers* (New York: Little, Brown, and Company, 2013), 72.

49 **an absolute fallacy:** Ibid.

Chapter Four

65 **competitors like Sara Lee:** For a fuller account of Grupo Bimbo, see Aaron Bobrow-Strain, *White Bread: A Social History of the Store-Bought Loaf* (Boston: Beacon Press, 2012), 153–55.

Chapter Five

68 **attributes the digestibility:** Jade Doyle, "3 Reasons Einkorn May Be Easier to Digest Than Other Types of Wheat," at http://www.einkorn.com/3-reasons-einkorn-may-be-easier-to-digest-than-other-types-of-wheat/.

69 **forty-two chromosomes in total:** "Why Is the Wheat Genome So Complicated?" at http://coloradowheat.org/2013/11/why-is-the-wheat-genome-so-complicated/.

69 **all agricultural crops:** Data compiled from http://coloradowheat.org/2013/11/why-is-the-wheat-genome-so-complicated/ and from Cold Spring Harbor Laboratory, http://www.cshl.edu/Article-McCombie/bread-wheats-large-and-complex-genome-is-revealed.

74 **adjusted in blending:** Data from http://www.faculty.ucr.edu/~legneref/botany/majcerea.htm; http://www.smallgrains.org/WHFACTS/6classwh.htm; and USDA Bulletin 1074 at http://

www.sustainablegrains.org/sitebuildercontent/sitebuilderfiles/clarkusdabulletin1074cat87212876.pdf.

76 **according to one historian:** Kevin Greene, "Technological Innovation and Economic Progress in the Ancient World: M. I. Finley Re-Considered," *Economic History Review* New Series 53, no. 1 (February 2000): 29–59.

76 **ten thousand and thirty thousand inhabitants:** Henry Cleere, *Southern France: An Oxford Archaeological Guide* (New York: Oxford University Press, 2001), 119–20. Other accounts triple the population estimate.

77 **"by his profession":** Quoted in Katherine Czapp, "The Case for Rejecting or Respecting the Staff of Life," *Against the Grain*, July 16, 2006, at http://maninisglutenfree.wordpress.com/2011/07/05/the-history-of-how-wheat-became-toxic. Her article contains a wealth of historical information and a spirited assault on industrialized wheats, "feats of mechanical and chemical engineering that are breathtaking in their sheer contempt for the art of traditional food preparation."

78 **by chewing wheat:** John Marchant, Bryant Reuben, and Joan Alcock, *Bread: A Slice of History* (Gloucestershire, UK: The History Press, 2008), 18.

Chapter Six

82 **"only as a ruin":** William C. Edgar, *The Medal of Gold* (Minneapolis, Minn.: The Bellman Company, 1925), 101–2.

84 **"also directly harmful":** Charles Edward Shelly, "Millstone Flour and National Nutrition," *British Medical Journal* 1, no. 3305 (May 3, 1924), 798–99, at http://www.ncbi.nlm.nih.gov/pmc/articles/PMC2304305/.

84 **white flour and sugar:** Michael Pollan, *Cooked: A Natural History of Transformation* (New York: The Penguin Press, 2013), 259–60.

85 **running on empty:** Aaron Bobrow-Strain, *White Bread: A Social History of the Store-Bought Loaf* (Boston: Beacon Press, 2012), 110–12.

86 **and folic acid:** Henry A. Schroeder, "Loss of Vitamins and Trace Minerals Resulting from Processing and Preservation of Foods," *American Journal of Clinical Nutrition* 24 (May 1971): 562–73.

86 **"dead of malnutrition":** Theodore R. Hazen, http://www.angelfire.com/journal/millbuilder/boulting.html.

87 **riboflavin (429 percent):** https://www.usaemergencysupply.com/information_center/using_whole_grain_foods/nutritional_content_of_whole_wheats_baking_flour.htm#.U8v6MlZzN0Q.

Chapter Seven

93 **crop since 1989:** http://www.foxbusiness.com/markets/2014/07/11/report-kansas-wheat-production-estimates-lowered-as-harvest-expected-to-show/ and http://www.sciencedaily.com/releases/2014/07/140710094340.htm.

96 **"new breeding trait":** Hetty C. van den Broeck et al., "Presence of Celiac Disease Epitopes in Modern and Old Hexaploid Varieties: Wheat Breeding May Have Contributed to Increased Prevalence of Celiac Disease," *Theoretical and Applied Genetics* 121, no. 8 (November 2010): 1527–39.

99 **"super gluten" theories:** Donald D. Kasarda, "Can an Increase in Celiac Disease Be Attributed to an Increase in the Gluten Content of Wheat as a Consequence of Wheat Breeding?" *Journal of Agricultural and Food Chemistry* 61, no. 6 (February 13, 2013): 1155–59.

101 **the Rockefeller Foundation:** A lifelong friend of Borlaug, Noel Vietmeyer, has documented his life and achievements in several books. Among them, *Our Daily Bread* (Lorton, Va.: Bracing Books, 2011) from which much of this profile is drawn. In *Against the Grain* (New York: North Point Press, 2004), Richard Manning argues that the Green Revolution's approach to agriculture was the first step in its dehumanization.

101 **"talk to me":** E. J. Kahn, "The Staffs of Life," *New Yorker*, November 12, 1984, 86.

103 **"eat their fill":** http://www.nytimes.com/2010/12/16/opinion/16iht-eddikotter16.html?_r=0 and Manning, *Against the Grain*, 71.

106 **"than any known":** Vietmeyer, *Our Daily Bread*, Kindle e-book, Location 8574.

107 **"people by 1980":** http://reason.com/blog/2009/09/13/norman-borlaug-the-man-who-sav.

107 **"kill each other":** http://www.npr.org/template/story/story.php?storyid=130734134.

108 **"habits and superstitions":** Henry J. Miller, "Norman Borlaug: Genius Behind the Green Revolution," *Forbes*, January 18, 2012, 1.

108 **"well camouflaged bureaucracy":** Roland Bailey, "The Man Who Saved More Lives Than Any Other Has Died," September 13, 2009, at http://reason.com/blog/2009/09/13/norman-borlaug-the-man-who-sav.

109 **6,000 pounds per acre:** Miller, "Norman Borlaug."

109 **self-sufficient in food:** "Ears of Plenty," *Economist* print edition, December 20, 2005, 7, at www.economist.com/node/5323362.

109 **"who has ever lived":** Gregg Easterbrook, "Forgotten Benefactor of Humanity," *Atlantic*, January 1, 1997, at http://www.theatlantic.com/magazine/archive/1997/01/forgotten-benefactor-of-humanity/306101/2/. Easterbrook wrote in the *Atlantic* that Borlaug was "the man who saved more human lives than any other person who ever lived."

111 **"deny them these things":** John Tierney, "Greens and Hunger," *New York Times*, May 19, 2008. Also quoted at http://en.wikipedia.org/wiki/Norman_Borlaug.

111 **the following year:** Ibid., an excellent overview of Borlaug's life and contributions.

112 **only 4 percent:** http://opinionator.blogs.nytimes.com/2014/04/09/a-green-revolution-this-time-for-africa/.

113 **genetically modified organisms:** http://blogs.ei.columbia.edu/2013/07/30/the-intensifying-debate-over-genetically-modified

-foods/ and http://www.thenation.com/blog/176863/twenty-six -countries-ban-gmos-why-wont-us#.

Chapter Eight

117 **"seems to kill it":** Sara Deseran, "The Grain of Truth," *San Francisco*, August 2013, 76–77, continued on 86–89. Deseran compares a Bay Area whole-grain think tank led by Bob Klein, owner of Oakland's Community Grains, to the culinary equivalent of Marvel Avengers in her comprehensive, energetic, and entertaining overview of the local whole-grain movement. Among the think tank's members are Chad Robertson, owner of famed Tartine Bakery in San Francisco and, of course, Craig Ponsford.

127 **eat those foods:** David R. Jacobs Jr. and Daniel D. Gallaher, "Whole Grain Intake and Cardiovascular Disease," *Current Atherosclerosis Reports*, November 6, 2004, 415–23.

127 **in the refining process:** http://www.health.state.mn.us/divs/hpcd /chp/cdrr/nutrition/docsandpdf/wholegrainfactsheet.pdf.

127 **the bottom rungs:** http://www.whfoods.com/genpage.php? tname=george&dbid=81.

127 **suggested daily total:** Anne Harding, "Fewer Than 1 in 20 in U.S. Eat Enough Whole Grains," Reuters, October 8, 2010, at http:// www.reuters.com/article/2010/10/08/us-whole-grains-idUSTRE69756N20101008.

128 **anti-inflammatory functions:** S. M. Kuo, "The Interplay Between Fiber and the Intestinal Microbiome in the Inflammatory Response," *Advances in Nutrition* 4, no. 1 (January 1, 2013): 16–28, at http://www.ncbi.nlm.nih.gov/pubmed/23319119.

128 **to asthma attacks:** http://www.jwatch.org/na33813/2014/03/04 /are-dietary-fiber-gut-microbiome-and-asthma-connected#sthash .d0VSfSME.dpuf.

130 **"leaves much to be desired":** Robert Lustig, *Fat Chance* (New York: Hudson Street Press, 2012), 130–33.

Chapter Nine

132 **points out in "Stone Soup":** Elizabeth Kolbert, "Stone Soup," *New Yorker*, July 28, 2014, 26–29.

133 **only one mile:** Ibid.

138 **chefs in 2013:** http://podbay.fm/show/602624887/e/1360938858?autostart=1.

Chapter Ten

151 **"straight in the oven":** Quoted in Andrew Whitley, *Bread Matters* (Kansas City, Mo.: Andrews McMeel Publishing, LLC, 2009), 119.

154 **"in the *miches*":** Ibid., 155.

Chapter Eleven

161 **opposite point of view:** Jared Diamond, "The Worst Mistake in the History of the Human Race," *Discover*, May 1987, 64–66.

172 **Jacobs and his team reported:** David R. Jacobs Jr. and Daniel D. Gallaher, "Whole Grain Intake and Cardiovascular Disease," *Current Atherosclerosis Reports*, November 6, 2004, 415–23.

176 **gluten-sensitive individuals:** O. Molber et al., "Mapping of Gluten T-Cell Epitopes in the Bread Wheat Ancestors: Implications for Celiac Disease," *Gastroenterology* 128, no. 2 (February 2005): 393–401, at http://www.ncbi.nlm.nih.gov/pubmed/15685550.

178 **process hulled wheats:** Emmer, not einkorn, is technically the ancestor of today's wheat.

179 **"highly immunoreactive gliadin":** The ∞/ ß-gliadin peptide.

Chapter Twelve

181 **system is struggling:** In conversation with the author. For an illuminating, well-researched, and highly recommended article by Jerry Adler, see "Artisanal Wheat on the Rise," *Smithsonian Magazine*, December 2011, which profiles Rogosa and some of

artisanal wheat's leadinging adherents. At http://www.smithsonianmag.com/arts-culture/artisanal-wheat-on-the-rise-85474/?all.

Chapter Thirteen

191 **don't eat much:** Nancy Harmon Jenkins, "From Italy, the Truth About Pasta; The Italians Know That Less Is More: A Call for a Return to Basics," *New York Times*, September 17, 1997, at http://www.nytimes.com/1997/09/17/dining/italy-truth-about-pasta-italians-know-that-less-more-call-for-return-basics.html.

193 **one scientific study reports:** H. van den Broeck et al., "In Search of Tetraploid Wheat Accessions Reduced in Celiac Disease–Related Gluten Epitopes," *Molecular BioSystems* 6, no. 11 (November 6, 2010): 2206–13.

194 **create loaf volume:** P. R. Shewry et al., "The Structure and Properties of Gluten: An Elastic Protein from Wheat Grain," *Philosophical Transactions of the Royal Society of London B Biological Sciences* 357, no. 1418 (February 28, 2002): 133–42, at http://www.ncbi.nlm.nih.gov/pubmed/11911770.

194 **network of molecules:** http://www.glycemicindex.com/faqsList.php#12http://www.glycemicindex.com/faqsList.php#12.

195 **feeling of satiation:** Christopher Wanjek, "The Dish on Pasta: Maligned Food Actually a Healthy Carb," *LiveScience*, July 26, 2012, at http://www.livescience.com/21851-maligned-pasta-good-carb.html.

196 **"what's in the food":** Andrew Curry, "Gluten-Free Dining in Italy," *New York Times*, June 26, 2014, at http://www.nytimes.com/2014/06/29/travel/gluten-free-dining-in-italy.html.

199 **I learned from Serventi and Sabban:** Silvano Serventi and Françoise Sabban, *Pasta: The Story of a Universal Food* (New York: Columbia University Press, 2002), 189.

200 **author of *Bet the Farm*:** Frederick Kaufman, *Bet the Farm* (Hoboken, N.J.: John Wiley & Sons, 2012), 229.

Chapter Fourteen

214 **thousands of converts:** Matthew Boyle, "Gluten Takes a Beating from Fad Dieters and Grain Giants," *Bloomberg*, November 12, 2013, at http://www.bloomberg.com/news/2013-11-12/grain-giants-go-gluten-free-to-plump-profits-on-fad-diet.html.

214 **5 percent of it whole:** "NAMA Issues First Flour Output Data; Decrease of About 3 % Indicated," *Milling and Baking News*, December 27, 2011, 18–19.

Chapter Fifteen

218 **confirmed the findings:** S. M. Stenman et al., "Enzymatic Detoxification of Gluten by Germinating Wheat Proteases: Implications for New Treatment of Celiac Disease," *Annals of Medicine* 41, no. 5 (May 2009): 390–400, at http://www.ncbi.nlm.nih.gov/pubmed/19353359.

219 **In the Mideast:** Katherine Czapp, "The Case for Rejecting or Respecting the Staff of Life," *Against the Grain*, July 16, 2006, at http://www.westonaprice.org/modern-diseases/against-the-grain/.

220 **no intestinal lining deterioration:** Carlo G. Rizzello et al., "Highly Efficient Gluten Degradation by Lactobacilli and Fungal Proteases During Food Processing: New Perspectives for Celiac Disease," *Applied and Environmental Microbiology* 73, no. 14 (July 2007): 4499–4507, at http://www.ncbi.nlm.nih.gov/pmc/articles/PMC1932817/.

224 **"associated with obesity":** Joseph M. Mercola, "'Good Gut Bacteria' May Help Fight Obesity," Mercola.com, June 18, 2011, at http://articles.mercola.com/sites/articles/archive/2011/06/18/good-gut-bacteria-may-help-fight-obesity.aspx.

229 **suitable temperature range:** Debra Wink, "Lactic Acid Fermentation in Sourdough," thefreshloaf.com, January 19, 2009, at http://www.thefreshloaf.com/node/10375/lactic-acid-fermentation-sourdough.

Chapter Sixteen

231 **unique Flatbush accent:** Patricia Gadsby and Eric Weeks, "The Biology of . . . Sourdough," *Discover*, September 3, 2003, at http://discovermagazine.com/2003/sep/featscienceof.

234 **"intolerance in humans":** Raffaella Di Cagno et al., "Sourdough Bread Made from Wheat and Nontoxic Flours and Started with Selected Lactobacilli Is Tolerated in Celiac Sprue Patients," *Applied and Environmental Microbiology* 70, no. 2 (February 2004): 1088–96.

236 **"positions in life":** Katherine Czapp, "The Case for Rejecting or Respecting the Staff of Life," *Against the Grain*, July 16, 2006, at http://www.westonaprice.org/modern-diseases/against-the-grain/7/16/06.

237 **must be at work:** Siri Carpenter, "That Gut Feeling," American Psychological Association 43, no. 8 (September 2012): 50, at http://www.apa.org/monitor/2012/09/gut-feeling.aspx.

References

The History of Wheat, Bread, and Milling

Belasco, W. "Food and the Counterculture: A Story of Bread and Politics." In *The Cultural Politics of Food and Eating: A Reader*, ed. James L. Watson and Melissa Caldwell, pp. 217–34. Malden, Mass.: Blackwell Publishing, 2005.

Bobrow-Strain, Aaron. *White Bread: A Social History of the Store-Bought Loaf*. Boston: Beacon Press, 2012. Valuable for his deeply researched history and enlightening commentary on its effects on our culture as well as our eating habits and nutrition.

Deutsch, Ronald M. *The New Nuts Among the Berries*. Palo Alto, Calif.: Bull Publishing Co., 1977. Deutsch's nuts—as in nutty individuals—include Sylvester Graham and John Harvey Kellogg.

Diamond, Jared. *Guns, Germs, and Steel*. New York: W. W. Norton, 1997.

Jacob, H. E., and Peter Reinhart (Intro). *Six Thousand Years of Bread*. New York: Skyhorse Publishing, 2007. Immensely rich in information and equally idiosyncratic. John Milton and a host of others show up in full glory.

Kahn, E. J. *The Staffs of Life*. Boston: Little, Brown & Co., 1985. Before Michael Pollan, Kahn was exploring the secret life of potatoes and grain seeds and such—not with equal insight, perhaps, but with impressive research and knowledge.

Kaufman, Frederick. *Bet the Farm: How Food Stopped Being Food.* Hoboken, N.J.: John Wiley and Sons, 2012.

Lawson, Publius. *The Invention of the Roller Flour Mill.* Charleston, S.C.: Nabu Press, 2010. Paperback reprint for 1923 hardcover.

Mann, Charles. *Uncovering the New World Columbus Created.* New York: Knopf, 2011. Includes a chapter on how wheat traveled to the New World.

Manning, Richard. *How Agriculture Has Hijacked Civilization.* New York: North Point Press, 2004. Manning picks up a theme that Diamond explores in *Guns, Germs, and Steel.*

Marchant, John, Bryan Reuben, and Joan Alcock. *Bread: A Slice of History.* Gloucestershire, UK: The History Press, 2008. The English perspective, academic and British in tone and substance.

Morgan, Dan. *Merchants of Grain: The Power and Profits of the Five Companies at the Center of the World's Grain Supply.* New York: The Viking Press, 1979.

Pennefeather, Shannon. *Mill City: A Visual History of the Minneapolis Mill District (Minnesota).* Minneapolis: Minnesota Historical Society, 2003. A chapter on flour milling.

Rees, Jonathan. *Industrialization and the Transformation of American Life: A Brief Introduction.* Armonk, N.Y.: M. E. Sharpe, 2013. Contains information on the Washburn A Flour Factory, the home of General Mills.

Rubel, William. *Bread: A Global History.* London: Reaktion Books, 2011. Short, part of Reaktion's Edible series, and filled with fifty-five color illustrations. Rubel, a food historian, knows his subject, crumb and crust alike.

Servenri, Silvano, and Françoise Sabban. *Pasta: The Story of a Universal Food.* New York: Columbia University Press, 2002.

Shprintzen, Adam D. *The Vegetarian Crusade: The Rise of an American Reform Movement, 1817–1921*. Chapel Hill: University of North Carolina Press, 2013. An academic, sober look back at some colorful characters, 1817–1921, including Graham, Bernarr Macfadden, and the feuding Kellogg brothers.

Wright, Clifford A. *A Mediterranean Feast*. New York: William Morrow and Company, 1999. I recommend Wright's book to anyone interested in food, the Mediterranean, plant taxonomy, European culture, or cooking—there are more than five hundred recipes in a book that isn't a cookbook. It is a feast in itself, about eight hundred pages long, oversized, ambitious, and outrageously knowledgeable on the origin and preparation of foods including bread and macaroni, a.k.a. dried pasta.

Bread and Baking

Alexander. William. *52 Loaves: A Half-Baked Adventure*. Chapel Hill, N.C.: Algonquin Books, 2011. A humorous home bread baker's memoir in search of what else?—the perfect loaf.

Deseran, Sara. "The Grain of Truth." *San Francisco*, August 5, 2013. An energetic and informative profile of the Bay Area's best artisan bakers, and a strong argument for not giving up your love of great breads to chase a gluten-free fad.

Glezer, Maggie. *Artisan Baking*. New York: Artisan, 2000. One of the first, and still informative. Glezer visits stone mills and Kansas wheat fields. Excellent sourdough recipes, too.

Hamelman, Jeffrey. *Bread: A Baker's Book of Techniques and Recipes*. Hoboken. N.J.: John Wiley and Sons, 2013. A detailed and exceptional guide, filed with a lifetime of knowledge. Hamelman is King Arthur Flour's resident bread guru.

Lahey, Jim. *My Bread: The Revolutionary No-Work, No-Knead Method*. New York: W. W. Norton, 2009.

McGee, Harold. *On Food and Cooking: The Lore and Science of the Kitchen*. New York: Scribner's, 1984. A great food writer's classic, with an encyclopedic reach and grasp of all things edible, wheat and bread included.

O'Brien, Keith. "Should We All Go Gluten-Free?" *New York Times Magazine*, November 25, 2011.

Pollan, Michael. *Cooked: A Natural History of Transformation*. New York: The Penguin Press, 2013. Food writing at its best—graceful, incisive, entertaining, and shot through with the author's passionate conviction that good whole food is a necessity, not a luxury, for us all. The two relevant sections are on fermentation and bread.

Reinhart, Peter. *The Bread Baker's Apprentice: Mastering the Art of Extraordinary Bread*. Berkeley, Calif.: Ten Speed Press, 2001.

———. *Bread Revolution: World-Class Baking with Sprouted and Whole Grains, Heirloom Flours, and Fresh Techniques*. Berkeley, Calif.: Ten Speed Press, 2014.

———. *Whole Grain Breads: New Techniques, Extraordinary Flavors*. Berkeley, Calif.: Ten Speed Press, 2007. Reinhart is an engaging writer as well as superb guide to making fabulous whole-grain breads.

Robertson, Chad. *Tartine Book No. 3: Modern Ancient Classic Whole*. San Francisco: Chronicle Books, 2013. Heritage grain brought up to date.

———. *Tartine Bread*. San Francisco: Chronicle Books, 2010. An instant classic.

Whitley, Andrew. *Bread Matters*. Kansas City, Mo.: Andrews McMeel Publishing, 2006. Vastly informative, passionately felt, and warmly instructive.

Heritage and Heirloom Wheats

Adams, Case. "The Fermentable Fiber Revolution." *Nutraceuticals World*, November 1, 2012. At www.nutraceuticalsworld.com.

Adler, Jerry. "Artisanal Wheat on the Rise." *Smithsonian Magazine*, December 2011. Highly recommended. At www.smithsonian mag.com.

Denn, Rebekah. "Baking with Unusual Wheats." Undated. www .sunset.com. Denn, writing for the *Sunset Magazine* website, visits the Bread Lab at Washington State University and delivers an excellent overview of heritage and ancient grains in the kitchen.

Donnelly, Kristin. "Best Heirloom Wheat Producers." October 2013. At www.foodandwine.com.

"Heritage Grains Making a Comeback." *Nutraceuticals World*, November 1, 2012. At www.nutraceuticalsworld.com.

Jenny (no last name). "Good Questions: Einkorn, Spelt, Emmer, Farro and Heirloom Wheat." February 10, 2014. At www.nour ishedkitchen.com. A quick overview, worth a look.

Scott, Stephen. "What's Wrong with Our Wheat?" May 23, 2013. At www.underwoodgardens.com.

Sen, Indrani. "Flour That Has the Flavor of Home." *New York Times*, September 10, 2008.

Simpson, Sarah, and Heather McLeod. *Uprisings: A Hands-On Guide to the Community Grain Revolution*. Gabriola Island, BC: New Society Publishers, 2013.

Health and Nutrition

Braly, James, and Ron Hoggan. *Dangerous Grains*. New York: Avery Press, 2002. One of the earliest anti-gluten books.

Brody, Jane. *Jane Brody's Nutrition Book: A Lifetime Guide to Good Eating for Better Health and Weight Control*. New York: Bantam Books, 1982. The *New York Times* columnist's chapter on fiber is still relevant, as is her advice on just about everything we eat.

Cox, Stan. "The Great Gluten Panic." Part 1, January 30, 2014. Part 2, February 6, 2014. At www.motherearth.news. Cox, a senior scientist at The Land Institute in Salina, Kansas, and former USDA wheat geneticist, is immensely informed. This two-part series is essential reading for anyone interested in separating fact from fiction about gluten. He makes a strong case for eating whole grains.

Czapp, Katherine. "Against the Grain." July 16, 2006. At Weston A. Price website, http://www.westonaprice.org/modern-diseases/against-the-grain/.

Jacobs, D. R., Jr., et al. "Whole-Grain Consumption Is Associated with a Reduced Risk of Noncardiovascular, Noncancer Death Attributed to Inflammatory Diseases in the Iowa Women's Health Study." *American Journal of Clinical Nutrition* 85 (2007): 1606–14.

Lustig, Robert H. *Fat Chance*. New York: Hudson Street Press, 2013. In case anyone still doubts that sugar wrecks us, Lustig confirms your worst fears while vividly charting food contents, explaining the digestive system and laying the case for fiber as a necessity.

Nestle, Marion. *What to Eat: An Aisle-by-Aisle Guide to Savvy Food Choices and Good Eating*. New York: North Point Press, 2006. Nestle, supremely knowledgeable, separates wheat from chaff; Pollan called it an indispensable guide. She takes a long, clear look at the health-related issues around commercial bread and labeling.

Roach, Mary. *Gulp*. New York: W. W. Norton and Company, 2013. Nobody does offensive subjects with more style and humor that Roach, including passing gas and other adventures along a scenic tour of the alimentary canal that winds its way to the Las Vegas home of gut-impacted Elvis Presley's former physician.

Spiller, Monica, and Gene Spiller. *What's with Fiber?* Laguna Beach, Calif.: Basic Health Publications, 2005. Spiller, the doyenne of California heritage wheat, and her late husband, a physician, explore the benefits of a plant-based, high-fiber diet.

Taubes, Gary. *Good Calories, Bad Calories: Fats, Carbs, and the Controversial Science of Diet and Health*. New York: Anchor Books, 2008. Taubes takes on sugar, starch, and empty carbs, with chapters on insulin and fiber.

Sourdough Science

Arendt, Elke K., Liam A. M. Ryan, and Fabio Dal Bello. "Impact of Sourdough on the Texture of Bread." *Food Microbiology* 24 (April 2007): 165–74.

Di Cagno, Raffaella, et al. "Sourdough Bread Made from Wheat and Nontoxic Flours and Started with Selected Lactobacilli Is Tolerated in Celiac Sprue Patient." *Applied and Environmental Microbiology* 70, no. 2 (February 2004): 1088–96.

Di Cagno, R., et al. "Pasta Made from Durum Wheat Semolina Fermented with Selected Lactobacilli as a Tool for a Potential Decrease of the Gluten Intolerance." *Journal of Agricultural and Food Chemistry* 53, no. 11 (June 1, 2005): 4393–402.

Gänzle, Michael G., et al. "Carbohydrate, Peptide and Lipid Metabolism of Lactic Acid Bacteria in Sourdough." *Food Microbiology* 24, no. 2 (2007): 128–38.

Gänzle, Michael G., et al. "Modeling of Growth of *Lactobacillus sanfranciscensis and Candida milleri* in Response to Process Parameters of Sourdough Fermentation." *Applied and Environmental Microbiology* 64, no. 7 (July 1998): 2616–23.

Gobbetti, Marco, et al. "Sourdough Lactobacilli and Celiac Disease." *Food Microbiology* 24, no. 2 (April 2007): 187–96.

Gobbetti, Marco, et al. "The Sourdough Fermentation May Enhance the Recovery from Intestinal Inflammation of Celiac Patients at the Early Stage of Gluten-Free Diet." *European Journal of Nutrition* 51, no. 4 (February 2, 2012): 507–12.

MacGuire, James. "Pain au Levain." *The Art of Eating*, no. 83 (Winter 2009). Technical details of making a levain starter.

Rizzello, C. G., et al. "Highly Efficient Gluten Degradation by Lactobacilli and Fungal Proteases During Food Processing: New Perspectives for Celiac Disease." *Applied and Environmental Microbiology* 73, no. 14 (July 2007): 4499–507.

Sugihara, T. F., L. Kline, and M. W. Miller. "Microorganisms of the San Francisco Sour Dough Bread Process." *Applied Microbiology* 21, no. 3 (March 1971): 456–58.

Wing, Daniel, and Alan Scott. *The Bread Builders*. White River Junction, Vt.: Chelsea Green Publishing Company, 1999. See "Baker's Resource: Sourdough Microbiology," p. 230.

Wink, Debra. "Lactic Acid Fermentation in Sourdough." January 19, 2009. At www.thefreshloaf.com. Wink's chemical analysis breaks down a complex subject and makes it accessible. Contrary to myth, the species that grow in sourdough starters, she reports, are not tied to geographic location but rather to the traditional practices in the different regions.

Index